Contents

Go to our website:
www.hardchoices.com
to find

Acknowledgments

Links to resources and help with
the topics in this book

Links to most of the references
found in the Endnotes

Information on purchasing copies of:
Hard Choices for Loving People
In English, Spanish, and Chinese
and
Light in the Shadows:
Meditations While Living with a Life-Threatening Illness
by Hank Dunn

About the Author

Since 1983, Hank Dunn has been ministering to patients at the end of their lives and their families. He served as a nursing home chaplain at Fairfax Nursing Center and as a staff chaplain for the Hospice of Northern Virginia, now Capital Hospice.

Hank is a graduate of the University of Florida and received his Master of Divinity degree from the Southern Baptist Theological Seminary in Louisville, Kentucky. After serving 5 years as a youth minister at a very traditional church in Macon, Georgia, he moved to the DC area to be a part of the very nontraditional Church of the Saviour. He worked a year as a carpenter and for 4 years directed an inner city ministry before moving into the chaplaincy in 1983.

He is a past president of the Northern Virginia Chapter of the Alzheimer's Association. He has served on the Ethics Committee at the Reston Hospital Center and the Chaplaincy Advisory Board at the Loudoun Hospital Center. He continues to volunteer as a chaplain at the Loudoun Hospital and at the Loudoun Adult Medical Psychiatric Services. For several years, Chaplain Dunn volunteered at Joseph's House, a home for formerly homeless men and women who are terminally ill. He is also a Volunteer Pastoral Associate at his faith community, Vienna Baptist Church, where he is especially involved in the retreat ministry at the Lost River Retreat Center in West Virginia.

To help him explain end-of-life decisions to patients and families, he wrote a booklet to hand to them so they could reflect on the issues discussed. As an afterthought, he sent the book out to other institutions to see if they would be interested in purchasing it for the people they serve. First published in 1990, *Hard Choices for Loving People* has sold over 2,000,000 copies, and is being used in more than 5,000 hospitals, nursing homes, faith communities, and hospice programs nationwide. His second booklet, *Light in the Shadows: Meditations While Living with a Life-Threatening Illness, Second Edition* was released in 2005. This is a collection of reflections on the emotional and spiritual concerns at the end of life.

Hank Dunn is a frequent speaker on topics related to the end of life.
He enjoys backpacking, kayaking, and hiking.

Fifth Edition

Hard Choices For Loving People

CPR,

Artificial Feeding,

Comfort Care,

and the Patient

with a

Life-Threatening

Illness

By Hank Dunn
Chaplain

Printing History

First Edition
September 1990-January 1992—93,979 (7 printings)

Revised Edition
April 1992-January 1994 —148,700 (8 printings)

Third Edition
July 1994-January 2001—589,163 (19 printings)

Fourth Edition
May 2001-September 2008—1,508,342 (21 printings)

Fifth Edition
June 2009—100,000
November 2009—10,000 (Spanish)
November 2009—3,500 (Chinese)
December 2009—100,000
June 2010—35,650
June 2010—10,000 (Spanish)
September 2010—59,438
March 2011—80,539
August 2011—83,693
October 2011—10,352 (Spanish)
December 2011—70,000

This book is published by:

A & A Publishers, Inc.

43608 Habitat Circle • Lansdowne, VA 20176-8254 • USA
Voice Mail - (571) 333-0169 • Fax - (571) 333-0167

Web site - www.hardchoices.com • *Email* - info@hardchoices.com
**Visit our Web site, write or call for information
on purchasing bulk copies.**

Cover photo of the Chesapeake Bay by Helmuth Humphrey
Cover design by Paul A. Gormont, Apertures, Inc., Sterling, VA

Introduction

On the occasion of her 102nd birthday, I went into Mable's room at the nursing home to ask her the secret to a long life. I expected some niceties like "clean living" or "just trust God," since she was a minister's wife. But she was too wise for that. "Mable, how do you live to be 102?" Without hesitation she responded, "Just keep breathing!" I wish it were so simple. If we want to stay alive, we "just keep breathing." Or when there is no hope of recovery from an illness, we could "just stop breathing." Real life is not so simple for patients in hospitals, nursing homes, or hospice programs, or for those who find themselves moving toward the end of a long decline in their health.

It is very important that patients and their families discuss the use of life-prolonging medical procedures.

Throughout most of our life, medical treatment decisions are quite simple. We get sick. Our doctor prescribes a treatment. Since we can only benefit from the physician's orders, we follow the treatment plan and return to our previous state of health. Yet as our health declines, medical decisions become more complex. Patients who have multiple medical problems, who are dependent on others for daily care like nursing home residents, or who have a terminal condition often face difficult treatment choices.

The difficulty arises from the fact that for patients with a life-threatening illness, or even a long-term chronic condition, some medical treatments offer little benefit. At the same time, these treatments may be painful or increase the burden of living. As we make decisions, we must constantly weigh possible benefits against possible burdens of a particular treatment plan. Sometimes people conclude that the burdens far outweigh any possible benefit and therefore refuse a particular treatment. Others feel that even a small potential benefit is worth the significant burdens.

The generations alive today are the first generations faced with making such difficult choices about potentially life-prolonging medical decisions. Modern medical developments like ventilators, feeding tubes, and cardiopulmonary resuscitation (CPR) have improved a few people's chances of surviving an accident, heart attack, or stroke. But the declining health of patients with multiple medical problems—and those with a terminal condition—make their outlook for survival much poorer than that of the general public. Therefore, it is very important that all patients with life-threatening illnesses and their families discuss the use of life-prolonging medical procedures.

The Four Most Common Decisions

This booklet is written to provide guidance to patients and their families who must face the "hard choices" as they receive and participate in healthcare. The "hard choices" are found in four questions that require treatment decisions[1] (1) Shall resuscitation be attempted? (pages 11-16); (2) Shall artificial nutrition and hydration be utilized? (pages 17-28); (3) Should a nursing home resident or someone ill at home be hospitalized? (pages 39-41); and (4) Is it time to shift the treatment goal from cure to hospice or comfort care only? (pages 29-38). Besides these four more common decisions, some attention will also be given to ventilators (breathing machines) (pages 41-43), dialysis (pages 43-44), antibiotics (pages 44-45) and pain control (pages 45-46) . Throughout this book, consideration will be given for how these treatments affect patients who are children or patients with dementia (for example, Alzheimer's). After a thoughtful reading of these pages, you may want to discuss what is contained here with your family and physician. The goal of this booklet is to give you enough information to help you make informed decisions.

Although I draw from my professional experience with these decisions, and I refer often to the medical research, I can only make general suggestions of treatment options one might consider. I recommend discussing medical treatments with your physician and other healthcare professionals familiar with your particular case. I can write only of my experiences with specific medical cases, and they may or may not be similar to the circumstances you are facing. All the stories I share are true, but, at times, I have changed names to protect privacy.

Goals of Medical Care

To begin thinking about potentially life-prolonging medical procedures it is first necessary to establish the intended goal of medical care.[2,3] The question is, "What outcome can we reasonably expect from medical treatment, given the current condition of the patient?" After the patient (or the decisionmaker for the patient) and the medical team agree on a goal, then the medical professionals can recommend ways to achieve that end.

Here are the three possible goals of medical care:

1. Cure. Almost all health care today is directed toward the prevention or cure of diseases. We become sick. The physician prescribes a treatment. We are cured.

2. Stabilization of functioning. Many disease processes cannot be cured, but medical treatment can stabilize the functioning of a patient or, in other words, temporarily stop the disease from getting worse. We have no cure for diabetes, but a person can take insulin injections for a lifetime and function fairly well. I knew a 32-year-old man with muscular dystrophy who breathed with the help of a mechanical ventilator. He used his voice-activated computer, was an avid sports fan, and had a great sense of humor. His treatment did not offer a cure, but he could function at a level acceptable to him. I have known several patients whose poorly functioning kidneys made it necessary for them to travel to a local hospital three times a week for dialysis. These treatments can be considered appropriate even though they offer no hope of cure.

3. Preparing for a comfortable and dignified death. This is the hospice, "comfort care only" or palliative care approach. Each of those same dialysis patients I just mentioned at one point decided that the treatment no longer offered them an acceptable quality of life, and so it was discontinued. They each died a short time later with appropriate care given to keep them comfortable. "Preparing for a comfortable and dignified death" is a shift in the focus and goals away from the direction of much of medical treatment given today. It is a shift away from most of the medical training our physicians receive. It is also a shift away from the mission of our hospitals, which exist primarily to cure patients.

At times, these goals can actually be combined. I have seen many people adopt a stance of "preparing for a comfortable and dignified death" in the face of their end-stage cancer, but choose to "cure" pneumonia with antibiotics. Others in similar circumstances decline even the antibiotics.

Goals often change as the patient's condition changes. I asked the man on the ventilator under what condition he would like it turned off so that he might be allowed to die a natural death. He said, "When I end up like my roommate, who makes no response to anyone."

One way to find out if a treatment can accomplish a hoped-for outcome is to try it for a little while. And one can try treatments for a period of time in an effort to cure or stabilize using what is called a "time-limited trial" and then reassess at the end of the trial (see page 27).

My first summer as a hospice chaplain I was reminded once again of the importance of setting goals first. We had admitted a new patient on a Friday. By the next Monday I had two urgent phone calls on my voice mail from a nurse and a social worker. They went something like this, "Hank, we have a new patient who is very close to dying and her daughter wants everything done to try and save her including CPR and ventilator support. Can you help?" The patient *What really makes these decisions "hard choices" has little to do with the medical, legal, ethical, or moral aspects of the decision process. The real struggles are emotional and spiritual.* indeed was very ill and it turned out she was within a week of dying regardless of her treatment choices. She was totally dependent on her daughter for her care. She had just been discharged from the hospital after they were able to get her off a ventilator. However, she still received her nutrition through a feeding tube.

When I got to the home, the patient was in a recliner chair in the middle of the family room. She could not speak or lift a hand, although she did listen and seemed to understand what was going on. At the end of my visit I asked the daughter to follow me out to the car so I could give her a copy of *Hard Choices*. I took the opportunity to try to convince her not to attempt heroic measures on her frail mother. We spoke for a while and soon, with tears running down her cheeks, she said, "All I want is for my mother to die peacefully here at home." I said, "We can help you with that, but it will not involve the rescue squad or putting your mother on machines."

I left. A few hours later, I received a call from the daughter. She had one question. "How long does it take a person to die if you stop artificial feeding?" I told her what my experience had been and assured her that we would keep her mother comfortable if she were to decide to stop the feedings. I had not brought up the thought of withdrawing the feeding tube. She had established the goal—"All I want is for my mother to die peacefully here at home." Then she could entertain the idea that perhaps a feeding tube is not compatible with a peaceful death. She did not have to make that decision because her mother did die peacefully at home three days later. Once she had the goal in mind, she could allow a peaceful death.

After establishing the goal, then the specifics of the treatments outlined in this booklet can be addressed.

In my nearly three decades as a nursing home, hospice and hospital chaplain, I have been at the bedsides of very ill patients, and I have discussed these choices with their families in the hall outside the patient's room. The content of this booklet comes not only from research but also from first-hand experience. I am convinced that what really makes these decisions "hard choices" has little to do with the medical, legal, ethical, or moral aspects of the decision process. The real struggles are emotional and spiritual. People wrestle with letting go and letting be. These are decisions of the heart, not just the head. In a final chapter I give my view on these decisions, especially on the spiritual and emotional struggles within.

Chapter *One*

Cardiopulmonary Resuscitation

This chapter will answer the following questions:
How successful are efforts to restart a heart?
Can we know ahead of time which patients are most likely not to be revived by resuscitation efforts?
How do patients let their wishes be known if they choose not to have resuscitation efforts?

During the 1960s, researchers developed a method of rescuing victims of "sudden death" called cardiopulmonary resuscitation (CPR). Basically, CPR is used when a person's heart and/or breathing stops. The rescuer applies force to the chest with the hands, thus compressing the heart, and breathes in the patient's mouth, filling the lungs with air. Thousands of lives are saved each year with CPR.

Originally, CPR was intended to be used for situations where death was accidental, such as drowning or electrical shock, or when an otherwise healthy person experienced a heart attack. Some of the early guidelines even went on to say that there were certain cases when CPR should not be used. "CPR is not indicated in certain situations, such as cases of terminal irreversible illness when death is not unexpected. . . . **Resuscitation in these circumstances may represent a positive violation of a person's right to die with dignity.**"[4] Today, in both hospitals and nursing homes, CPR has become standard procedure on all patients who experience heart or breathing failure except for those with orders restricting its use.

Survival Rates with CPR

If a hospital patient's heart stops, a "code" is called and a special team responds. Treatment may include CPR, electrical shock to the heart, injection of medications, and the use of a ventilator. Approximately 35 percent of hospital patients whose heart or breathing stops[5] and 3 percent of nursing home residents in a similar condition[6,7] receive resuscitation attempts.

Medical researchers reviewed 113 studies on the use of CPR in hospitals conducted over a 33-year period.[5] They found that of the 26,095 patients who received resuscitation attempts, 3,968 or 15.2 percent survived to be discharged from the hospital. Over the years these survival rates have remained the same.[8-11]

Patients with the least chance of survival (less than 2 percent survive):
- those who have more than one or two medical problems;
- those who do not live independently or, in other words, are dependent on others for their care or live in a long-term care facility like a nursing home; and
- those who have a terminal disease.[12]

CPR in Nursing Homes

Nursing homes have professionals on duty trained to administer CPR. If CPR is begun, the staff will call 911 and the rescue squad will arrive. Once on the scene, the paramedics take over the care of the resident. They will then continue CPR until the patient has been transported to the nearest emergency room, where the staff will do everything in their power to bring the patient back to life. Measures could include continuing CPR, electrical shock, or ventilators. Once in the emergency room, patients may be connected to mechanical devices to keep them breathing through a tube inserted in the mouth and down the windpipe.

Calling 911 means everything possible will be done to resuscitate the patient. We, as a community, need to know that the rescue squad will respond as quickly and as aggressively as possible to save lives.

The research on CPR in the nursing home indicates only 0-2 percent of the patients receiving resuscitation attempts survive. **Why does CPR offer so little hope of medical benefit for the frail, debilitated nursing home resident? Most of the characteristics that point to a poor prognosis for the survival in hospital patients are common in nursing home residents.**[13-16] By definition, residents do not live independently because of their generally failing health. Most have multiple medical problems.

Some people ask, "Can we just try CPR at the nursing home and not transfer a resident to the emergency room, where they do more aggressive treatment?" This is not standard procedure and for good reason. The professionals at a nursing home want as much support as possible if they are trying to revive a resident. That support can come only from a rescue squad, and only the advanced medical team at an emergency room can determine whether all attempts at reviving have failed. Once the chain of events is set in motion, it is very difficult to stop until every procedure has been attempted. If successfully revived, the patient will then need to be in the hospital for the follow-up care.

Burdens of CPR

Like most medical procedures, CPR does have some burdens. A frail patient's ribs could be broken and a lung or spleen punctured because of the necessary force applied during CPR. If too much time has elapsed since the patient has been without oxygen, there will be brain damage. The brain injury can range from subtle

Because of the chain of events put into motion when CPR is begun, a person could be placed on a breathing machine even though he or she might not have wanted it.

changes in intellect and personality all the way to permanent unconsciousness ("persistent vegetative state").[17] Because of the chain of events put into motion when CPR is begun, a person could be placed on a breathing machine even though he or she might not have wanted it. For many patients this risk of prolonged survival "on machines" with severe brain injury is a very serious burden. Also, CPR severely reduces the possibility of a peaceful death.

CPR and the Patient with a Life-Threatening Illness

Some patients may benefit from CPR.[5] A frank discussion with a physician will help any patient assess the possible benefit.

But those who find themselves among the "patients with the least chance of survival" group will find the medical benefits from CPR are minimal. Again, this would include (1) patients with multiple medical problems, (2) those who have a terminal disease, or (3) those who are dependent on others for care, including long-term nursing home residents. In deciding whether to accept or reject CPR, one must weigh the facts. **Once a patient with one of these conditions has a cardiac or respiratory arrest, there is only the smallest of possibilities of having the heart restarted and almost no chance of surviving the subsequent hospitalization.**

The frailty that goes with the worsened medical condition common among these patients contributes to this poor outlook for survival. Even if the patient survives the event that required CPR, the chances of long-term survival are slim and the individual's condition will most likely be much worse than before. Given these facts, many people choose not to have CPR used as a medical treatment. Others feel that CPR offers some hope of survival and that every effort should be made to save a person's life no matter the medical condition or prognosis.

CPR with Children

Age has not been shown to be a factor in the success of CPR. Some of the same conditions that make resuscitation attempts unsuccessful in the general population apply to children. Children with multiple organ system failure or those in the terminal phase of a disease have little chance of surviving CPR. What makes the decision to withhold resuscitation attempts on these little ones so difficult is the overwhelming sense of loss for the parents and for the medical staff. For a parent to say "do not resuscitate" symbolizes the lost future of the child and lost hopes of the parents. The physician and other healthcare workers can help sort out the "medical side" of this decision. The more difficult part is letting go.

CPR Is the Standard Order

Upon admission to a nursing home or hospital, it is assumed that every patient whose heart stops will receive CPR. This presumption *for* CPR is reasonable since any delay in beginning the procedure greatly reduces the chances for success. If a person would rather not have resuscitation attempts, a doctor must write an order restricting its use. This order goes by many different names: "No Code," "No CPR," "DNR" (do not resuscitate), "DNAR" (do not attempt resuscitation) or "AND" (allow natural death). This order must be given by the physician, and often the family or the patient must request it. In most cases the staff or physicians will not make a DNR decision without a discussion with the patient or family, no matter how seriously ill a patient may be.

It is also assumed when 911 is called that the rescue squad will try CPR on any person whose heart or breathing stops. Many states provide a document or bracelet to show the emergency personnel if the patient would not want to receive resuscitation attempts. Sometimes called an "Out-of-Hospital DNR Order," this paper can allow a family to feel confident in calling the rescue squad for help. They can know they will receive comfort care and supportive help for the patient while not running the risk of attempts at resuscitation or being "hooked up to machines."

Summary:

About 15 percent of patients in hospitals who have CPR attempts survive to be discharged.

Patients with multiple medical problems, with a terminal illness, or who cannot live independently survive CPR less than 2 percent of the time.

Possible burdens of "successful" CPR include the following: fractured ribs and punctured lungs, brain damage, depression, never regaining consciousness, risk of patient's remaining days connected to machines, and reduced possibility of a peaceful death

Patients, or those making decisions for them, may request from the physician an order not to attempt resuscitation.

Chapter *Two*

Artificial Hydration and Nutrition

> **This chapter will answer the following questions:**
> What are some of the benefits and hazards of artificial feeding tubes?
> What are some of the advantages of dying without the use of artificial feeding or IVs?
> What is a time-limited trial?

When a patient can no longer take food or fluid by mouth, a feeding tube can sometimes be used to overcome this disability. Tubes usually come in one of two types. The nasogastric (NG) tube is inserted through the nose, down the esophagus, and into the stomach. The gastrostomy is a tube inserted surgically through the skin into the stomach wall. Liquid nutritional supplements, water, and medications can be poured into the tube or pumped in by way of a mechanical device. Sometimes this method is called a PEG* tube. There is also the less common TPN**, when a catheter or needle is inserted in a vein, often in the chest, and a liquid containing nutrients is pumped directly into the blood stream, bypassing the digestive system.

Feeding tubes have proved beneficial to thousands of patients. Many people, such as some stroke patients, need the help of a feeding tube for a short period before going back to eating

---

*percutaneous endoscopic gastrostomy.
**total parenteral nutrition

by mouth. Others live with a gastrostomy tube and enjoy reading, watching television, or visiting with their families. I had one patient who had lost the ability to swallow due to throat cancer and had a feeding tube. He lived alone and was hampered in his ability to care for himself because of emphysema. I asked him once how he felt about the feeding tube. He said, "Great! I don't have to go grocery shopping. I don't have any pots and pans to wash. And I can stay in my own home." Clearly he felt he benefited from the feeding tube.

Feeding tubes have proved beneficial to thousands of patients.

Often, however, a patient with a life-threatening or long-term chronic illness never regains the ability to eat or drink. Some people survive for years on a feeding tube. Karen Ann Quinlan, although disconnected from a respirator, lived unconscious for more than 10 years receiving nutrition and hydration through a feeding tube. Rita Greene, who made no response to any stimuli, lived for 48 years with the aid of a feeding tube.[18]

Patients who make no sort of purposeful response to their surroundings have been variously described as permanently unconscious patients or patients in a persistent (or permanent) vegetative state (PVS).[19,20] Most often these patients suffered brain damage from an interruption of the flow of blood to the brain. All their vital body functions operate without the aid of machinery with only the artificially supplied hydration and nutrition needed to keep them alive. Frequently they are young people left in this condition after an automobile or sporting accident.

As one might expect, a variety of opinions are expressed on whether or not to artificially feed and/or hydrate hopelessly ill or dying patients. There is a wealth of research and opinions on the use of artificial hydration and nutrition with the goal of discovering whether or not using it is helpful to the patient or whether it does harm.[21-41]

Often the standard medical practice is to start tube feeding for any patient who can no longer take in enough food or water by mouth. A patient may receive a feeding tube unless the patient or family makes a conscious choice not to do so.

Intravenous (IV) Artificial Hydration

A common method of artificial hydration, especially in a hospital, is the IV line. Through a needle or plastic tube (catheter) in the arm, a patient can receive fluids and medications. The process of inserting the IV can be uncomfortable. The patient may have to have the point of insertion changed frequently if the IV does not work, or if 3-5 days have elapsed, to prevent infection or irritation. If patients pull at the tubes, their hands may need to be tied down. For most patients, these are appropriate and acceptable burdens.

Although this chapter mostly addresses the use of feeding tubes, IVs are related. When used to hydrate a dying patient, IVs are included in the discussion of artificial feeding tubes because they both supply hydration artificially. Patients and families should frequently reconsider whether the use of IVs is appropriate, especially as the time of death approaches. Much of what we know about withholding artificial hydration at the end of life has been discovered as caregivers observed patients dying with and without the use of IV fluids.

The Burdens of Artificial Feeding

Feeding tubes are not without risk. Pneumonia can develop if the tube becomes displaced or if regurgitated fluid (vomit) enters the lungs. Ulcers and infections can also result from a feeding tube. A patient who repeatedly removes the tube will probably need to be restrained by tied hands or sedation. The immobility of most of these patients makes them prime candidates for bedsores and a stiffening of the limbs from lack of movement.

Furthermore, patients can be more isolated with artificial feeding than hand feeding because they lose the personal interaction of someone sitting and feeding them three times a day. A stroke patient with an artificial feeding tube came to our nursing home from the hospital. She made some response to those who gave her care and to her family. The family had agreed they would try the feeding tube for a year and if there was no improvement, they would stop the treatment and let her die. At the end of the year, along with withdrawing the artificial feeding, a speech therapist worked with the patient to try to help her eat again by mouth. Not only did she live for another year without the artificial feeding, but her whole personality changed. She was more interactive, smiled more, and generally seemed to be in better health. I know this is just one case, but we were able to observe her with and without artificial feeding. I am convinced that the personal connection with a nurse or aide three times a day, plus just the pleasurable stimulation of eating, changed this woman's life.[42]

Patients can be more isolated with artificial feeding than hand feeding.

The Case for Artificial Feeding in All Circumstances

Some say that no matter what the prognosis for recovery, a feeding tube should always be used because food and water are basic human rights that should not be denied to anyone. Those who advocate such a position often allow that an adult who is able to make decisions can refuse any medical treatment, including artificial hydration and nutrition.

Those who advocate using a feeding tube under all circumstances often characterize the act of not providing hydration and nutrition artificially as "starvation." Indeed, anyone who does not receive food and water will die (though their condition would more accurately be described as "dehydrated" rather than "malnourished")[43,44] They describe the insertion of a feeding tube as just providing "basic food and water" like hand feeding and, therefore, not a medical intervention.[45] Additionally, since the patient will die in a short time if a feeding tube is removed, they may argue that the intent of those removing the tube is to end the life of the patient, which is clearly against the very nature of medicine.[46]

The Case Against Artificial Feeding in Some Circumstances

Many consider the use of artificial feeding tubes, in some cases, as causing excessive burdens, and we are not obligated to use them. Many say that artificial forced feeding of terminally ill persons or those in an irreversible coma is more of a burden than a benefit. Even though food and water are basic to our human existence, we are not obligated to replace the natural function of eating with an artificial method. People who choose not to have their life prolonged on a mechanical ventilator are "denied" air, and some consider feeding tubes to be the same type of invasion of the patient.

People who advocate the removal of feeding tubes in some circumstances see the inability to take in food and water by mouth as a terminal medical condition. To withhold or withdraw artificial feeding is to allow a natural death to occur.[47] When a person dies after the withholding of artificial food and fluids, the death is from the condition or disease that made the patient unable to eat, not from the removal of artificial feeding. Therefore, nothing is being introduced to "kill" the patient, but the natural process of dying is being allowed to progress.[48] Choosing not to force-feed a person is choosing not to prolong the dying process.

The American Medical Association (AMA), in March 1986, issued a statement acknowledging that a doctor can ethically withdraw all means of life-prolonging medical treatment, including food and water, from a patient in an irreversible coma. Courts in many states and the U.S. Supreme Court have upheld this view and allowed the withdrawal of feeding tubes. A consensus is forming among state legislatures and in the medical literature viewing artificial feeding as a medical procedure that may be withdrawn.[43,49,50]

Would Withholding or Withdrawing Artificial Feeding Cause a Painful Death?

To characterize death after the withholding or withdrawal of artificial hydration and nutrition as "starvation" (and therefore perhaps causing suffering) is inaccurate. The patient's condition would more correctly be described as dehydrated. Whatever pain or discomfort is associated with malnutrition (starvation) is not relevant here because a patient will be affected by dehydration long before suffering any ill effects from the lack of nutritional support. Therefore, the question of pain control must address any pain a dehydrating patient may suffer as well as addressing the relief of acute pain that may be the result of another condition, such as cancer.

A genuine concern on everyone's part is pain control. If a patient is allowed to die by forgoing artificial feeding, can pain and discomfort be held to a minimum? The answer is yes.

Patients who have had brain damage and no longer respond to their environment "cannot experience pain and suffering."[20] For patients who have some responses, **there are ways to alleviate acute pain without the use of artificial feeding tubes or IV hydration.**

Beyond the issue of acute pain is the question of whether dying of dehydration causes any other unnecessary pain or unusual suffering. **The medical evidence is quite clear that dehydration in the end stage of a terminal illness is a very natural and compassionate way to die.** [21-41]

The benefits of NOT using artificial hydration (for example, an IV or feeding tube) in a dying patient:

- less fluid in the lungs and, therefore, less congestion, making breathing easier;
- less fluid in the throat and, therefore, less need for suctioning;
- less pressure around tumors and, therefore, less pain;
- less urination and, therefore, less need to move the patient for changing the bed and less risk of bedsores;
- less fluid retained in the patient's hands, feet, and the whole body in general. Forcing liquids into a person whose body is shutting down can create an uncomfortable buildup of fluid.
- a natural release of pain-relieving chemicals as the body dehydrates. Some have even described it as "mild euphoria."[25] This state that comes with no food intake also suppresses appetite and causes a sense of well-being.

The only uncomfortable symptoms of dehydration are a dry mouth and a sense of thirst, both of which can be alleviated with good mouth care and ice chips or sips of water but are not necessarily relieved by artificial hydration.

No matter what the treatment choice regarding feeding tubes, comfort care and freedom from pain are essential goals of any medical team. Just because extraordinary or heroic measures have been withheld or withdrawn does not mean that routine nursing care and comfort care are withheld. A patient will always receive pain medication, oxygen, or any other treatment deemed necessary to ensure as much comfort as possible.

The Difference Between Withholding and Withdrawing

Imagine how emotionally difficult it would be to withdraw a feeding tube from a person who has been kept alive through artificial means for several months or years. For a family and physician to change the treatment plan like this requires a change in perspective. A person has been living with a feeding tube and now the decision has been made to allow that person to die. It is not impossible, emotionally, to come to this point of withdrawing treatment, but it is more difficult than withholding the artificial feeding in the first place.

From moral, ethical, medical, and most religious viewpoints there is no difference between withholding and withdrawing. Emotionally, there is a world of difference. And as much as we would like to think physicians do not make decisions and recommendations based on emotion, it is difficult for them to suggest or accept a change from using the tube to withdrawing. A family I once knew wanted to withdraw artificial feeding from the patient, and the physician told me, "I would have had no problem not starting the treatment in the first place but I cannot order the withdrawal." There is nothing in law, medicine, ethics, or morality to justify such a stance. If withholding treatment would have been acceptable earlier, then only emotion could now require its continuation.[39]

From moral, ethical, medical, and most religious viewpoints there is no difference between withholding and withdrawing. Emotionally, there is a world of difference.

The difficulty of making the decision to withdraw treatment makes it very important to think through and discuss these issues long before a crisis comes. **If a patient or family does not want to use artificial feeding, it is much better not to begin the feeding at all. But if it is begun, artificial feeding can be withdrawn at a later date.**

Artificial Feeding and the Dementia Patient

Alzheimer's disease and similar conditions are characterized by the deterioration of the person over a number of years. In earlier stages of the disease, it may be helpful to the patient to use a feeding tube as a temporary measure in the event of a decline in appetite or weight loss. The hope is that the patient will eventually be able to take in enough food and fluid by mouth to be able to discontinue the tube.

In advanced dementia, research has shown that a feeding tube does not offer benefit to the patient, even with temporary use. Dementia is a terminal disease. Like all terminal conditions, dementia has symptoms that indicate when the end of the disease process may be near.

One of the problems in the terminal phase of this disease may be swallowing difficulties that have sometimes been treated with feeding tubes. **The truth is artificial feeding does not lengthen the life of an end-stage dementia patient and only adds greater burdens.**[52]

The signs of the end-stage of dementia are well documented:[53-56]
- incontinence;
- progressive loss of speech;
- loss of intentional movement;
- complete dependence for dressing, eating, and toileting;
- inability to recognize loved ones;
- and finally, eating difficulties, possibly including the loss of the ability to swallow.

One of the main hazards of hand feeding is the possibility for the patient to get food in the lungs and risk getting aspiration pneumonia. Some would rather start an artificial feeding tube to try to avoid the difficulties of hand feeding while hoping to reduce the possibility of causing pneumonia. Careful hand feeding (for example, keeping the head of the bed elevated and using soft foods) can reduce, though not eliminate, this risk, but the risk is not eliminated by tube feedings either. Some research indicates that pneumonia is a greater risk with a feeding tube.[53]

Many physicians, and others in healthcare, feel that because the feeding tube does not lengthen the life of the patient and causes greater burdens, careful hand feeding should be continued and artificial feeding is not appropriate.[53,56-76] Although pneumonia is a risk, those who would forgo the feeding tube view it as an acceptable risk. **They see the swallowing difficulties as part of the end of a very tragic disease process and know that introducing artificial feeding does not cure the underlying affliction–dementia.**

In 1999, a review[63] of 77 studies conducted over 33 years found that tube feeding of advanced dementia patients offered absolutely no benefit and even caused some harm. The researchers concluded, "We identified no direct data to support tube feeding of demented patients with eating difficulties for any of the commonly cited indications." Several more recent studies have come to similar conclusions.[56,66-72,77]

The facts about tube feeding for advanced dementia patients (like end-stage Alzheimer's):

"Tube feeding is a risk factor for aspiration pneumonia.

Survival has not been shown to be prolonged by tube feeding.

Feeding tubes have not been shown to prevent or heal pressure sores (bedsores).

Improved delivery of nutrients via tube has not been shown to reduce infection, but on the contrary, feeding tubes have been shown to cause serious local and systemic infection.

Functional status has not been improved and demented patients are not more comfortable with tube feeding while dozens of serious adverse effects have been reported."[63]

Artificial Feeding and Children

As difficult as it may be to withhold or withdraw artificial feeding from a failing 80-year-old, it only gets harder in making a decision like this for a child. With elderly persons who have always fed themselves, we can usually accept the stopping eating as a sign that the end of life is near. But a child is just beginning life. The medical realities may be no different between the seriously ill child and the adult . . . but it feels different. Furthermore, we would not expect young children or infants to be able to feed themselves even if they were healthy. So artificial hydration and nutrition might be seen as just another way of helping them "eat." From the first hours of a child's life parents seek to feed their little ones. These are difficult feelings to overcome as one considers refusing artificial feeding.

Again, as with CPR, the grief issues are great. We are having to let go of our child, the child's future, our future, our hopes . . . all difficult things to do.

A Time-Limited Trial

Patients who are having eating difficulties, or their families, should at least consider several treatment options—to use or not to use artificial feeding tubes or to use a compromise treatment plan. One compromise option is a time-limited trial of a feeding tube.[1,34,65] To do this, secure an agreement with the attending physician to try artificial feeding for a limited time, and if there is little or no improvement in the patient, or no possibility of regaining consciousness or the ability to swallow, then the artificial feeding may be withdrawn. **Another compromise is using artificial feeding to supplement hand feeding.** I know some patients who eat what they can during the day and have a feeding tube running at night.

No matter whether you choose for or against a feeding tube, you can find plenty of company. Religious leaders, ethicists, politicians, nurses, and physicians are divided on this issue. If the patient cannot make the decision, the family will have to decide on behalf of the patient. They will have to live with their decision, which may be a difficult burden to carry. I am convinced that this burden is heavy because of the emotional/spiritual struggle of the family in letting go. Medicine, law, ethics, and morality all are affected by this emotional struggle. It is understandable that people struggle with this issue. We are letting go of someone important to us. Even when it makes perfect sense, from a medical viewpoint, to withhold or withdraw artificial feeding, it can still be hard. I discuss this emotional and spiritual struggle in more detail in the final chapter.

Summary:

Feeding tubes can help many patients get through temporary times of eating difficulties and other patients choose to use one permanently after they have lost the ability to swallow.

Permanently unconscious patients can be maintained for years with a feeding tube, but people disagree whether such treatment should be withdrawn.

Patients with advanced dementia (like end-stage Alzheimer's) will not be helped with the use of artificial feeding tubes and may actually be harmed.

A time-limited trial can be used to try a treatment for a period of time, and, if it does not help the patient, then it can be discontinued.

Dying patients are much more comfortable without the use of artificial hydration.

Chapter Three

Cure Sometimes–Comfort Always:
Hospice, Palliative Care, and the
"Comfort Care Only" Order

This chapter will answer the following questions:

When is the "right time" to "prepare for dying"?

What is hospice?

How can I try to assure that there will be a peaceful dying?

What is appropriate care for end-stage dementia patients?

How do we know when a medical procedure is making the dying process unnatural and burdensome or when it offers promise of cure or freedom from pain? How can we prepare for the death of someone we love and make the experience as meaningful and as pain free as possible? The hospice movement has led the way in answering these questions. It has taught us that letting someone die naturally does not mean we stop treating or caring for the patient.

Although enrolling in a hospice program offers wonderful benefits to the dying and their families, one can have the same treatment approach at home or in a hospital or nursing home without a hospice program. In a nursing home this approach is most commonly characterized by a physician's order called "comfort care only" or "palliative care only."[78-80]

Many hospitals have a "palliative care" program designed to provide comfort care at the end of life. To understand the meaning of this approach, it is helpful to review the goals of medical treatment.

The Goals of Medical Treatment in the "Last Phase of Life"

We have a real difficulty today answering the question, "When am I dying?" Up until the second half of the 20th century our final illness was usually short and it was clear that the patient would die within the foreseeable future. Nowadays most of us will die of chronic diseases such as heart disease, cancer, stroke, or dementia. We will probably live with these diseases for years before dying of them. We may have times of being very close to death, recover, and then live for months, if not years.[81]

In my work as a nursing home and hospice chaplain, I have found that rather than talking about "dying" I might

What about the last phase of life as we live with a long-term chronic illness?

ask, "Would you say your mother is in the last phase of her life?" For seriously ill patients, most people are comfortable referring to the illness as part of the "last phase" even though they may not say "dying." We usually reserve the term "dying" for the last hours or days of a person's life.

In the Introduction (pages 7-10) I described **the three possible goals of medical care as: 1. Cure. 2. Stabilization of functioning. 3. Preparing for a comfortable and dignified death.** Clearly, when we know a person has reached the final hours of life, almost all of us would choose "preparing for a comfortable and dignified death." Equally clear, when we are healthy and have no other medical problems, we would usually choose to "cure" an illness.

What about the last phase of life as we live with a long-term chronic illness? Well, sometimes we choose "cure" and sometimes "preparing for death." I have seen many patients with congestive heart failure who suffer a life-threatening episode rushed to the hospital for aggressive curative treatment. Sometimes, the very next day they are back at home resuming activities. So it is appropriate, in some cases, for heart patients to be hospitalized. But some of these patients get to the point when they or their family decides "no more hospitals." Fortunately, good medical care can offer an acceptable quality of life in the home even though the disease cannot be "cured."

At any point during an illness . . . patients and families need to prepare emotionally and spiritually for the possibility of death. This preparation can be accomplished even while aggressively treating symptoms.

At any point during a long-term chronic illness like heart failure, Alzheimer's, or respiratory failure, or during a more short-term illness like some cancers, patients and families need to prepare emotionally and spiritually for the possibility of death. This preparation can be accomplished even while aggressively treating symptoms that could bring death at any time. All during the course of the illness, patients and families need to weigh the benefits of treatment with the quality of life. If quality of life diminishes, some patients may opt to stop some treatment to preserve quality. The aggressive treatment no longer provides the benefit to the patient and the choice is made to "prepare for a comfortable and dignified death."

When asked, most people say, "I want to die peacefully in my sleep in my own bed." Sometimes, a few people have told me, "I would like to die in a hospital." The hope is that the patient's preference can be honored. For those who would like to die peacefully in their own home, hospice may be a good option.

Hospice

The term "hospice" (from the same linguistic root as "hospitality") can be traced back to early Western Civilization when it was used to describe a place of shelter and rest for weary or sick travelers on long journeys. The term was first applied to specialized care for dying patients in 1967, at St. Christopher's Hospice in a residential suburb of London."At the center of hospice is the belief that each of us has the right to die pain-free and with dignity, and that our families will receive the necessary support to allow us to do so. The focus is on caring, not curing and, in most cases, care is provided in the patient's home. Hospice also is provided in freestanding hospice facilities, hospitals, and nursing homes and other long-term care facilities."[82]

A hospice provides a team of professionals and specially trained volunteers to address the medical, social, psychological, and spiritual needs of the patient and the family. If the choice is made to stay at home, the hospice team is available 24 hours a day, 7 days a week, for support, consultation, and visits. In a hospital or nursing home, the team becomes an adjunct to the staff, advising, teaching, observing and supporting the patient and family, and providing extra equipment aids, if needed. Inpatient hospice facilities incorporate the whole hospice philosophy in a unique setting with specially trained staff. Wherever hospice serves, emphasis is on management of pain and other symptoms and quality of life rather than length of life.[83] Hospice care continues after

Wherever hospice serves, emphasis is on management of pain and other symptoms and quality of life rather than length of life.

a death with grief counseling services for both families and friends of the patient.

What Are Comfort Measures?

Some treatments are clearly intended to provide comfort to a patient and not prolong the dying process. For example, pain medication and medicines to help reduce a fever are comfort measures. Oxygen can be used to make breathing easier. Routine nursing care such as keeping the patient clean and dry and changing the linens and clothes adds to the comfort of the one who is dying. Emotional and spiritual support, both to the patient and the family, are provided by staff members, chaplains, and volunteers. Choosing hospice or "comfort care only" does not mean care or treatment stops. **"Cure sometimes–comfort always" is a constant reminder of the goals of this approach.**

Which Medical Treatments Are Optional?

A "comfort care only, " palliative care, or hospice approach may add some new comfort measures mentioned above. Some treatments might be withheld or withdrawn:

• Usually a cancer patient would no longer be receiving radiation or chemotherapy in an effort to cure the disease, but these methods might be used to relieve pain.

• Antibiotics may not routinely be used to treat an infection like pneumonia, but the patient may choose to seek a cure from it. Again, antibiotics may be used if necessary to relieve pain. (see pages 44-45)

• Most diagnostic testing may be eliminated, especially testing that might involve painful procedures like drawing blood. The reasoning here is that if there will no longer be active treatment to cure the patient, then diagnostic testing is not needed.

• A feeding tube would not routinely be started, but if one is already in place, then withdrawal of the tube could be considered separate from the "comfort measures only" order.

Remember, artificial hydration may only add to the discomfort of the dying patient. Likewise, IVs might be used as a means of infusing pain medication but usually not for hydration.

• Usually surgery would not be performed unless it was deemed absolutely necessary to promote the comfort of the patient.

Which Patients Are Candidates for Hospice or Comfort Care Only? When Is the Right Time?

Hospice care is used for those with a life-limiting progressive illness with 6 months or less to live if the disease runs its normal course. Often, but not always, hospice patients know that cure is impossible. They wish a high quality of life for however long they have left. **Early admission into a hospice program allows more time for the hospice team to fully understand the patient's and family's needs and to develop a suitable plan of care.** Perhaps most important of all, if a relationship of trust between patient and hospice can develop over several months, the patient enjoys the full benefit of hospice care.

Hospice care is used for those with a life-limiting progressive illness with 6 months or less to live if the disease runs its normal course.

Any person who is in the end-stage of any disease process would be a candidate for a "comfort care only" order and certainly for a hospice program. Of course, a patient with the capacity to make decisions may refuse any treatment with a goal of cure or stabilization and request a "comfort care only" order. Physicians and nurses can provide guidance to determine when a patient is probably in the end-stage of a disease.

It would be a mistake to say that on "one day" the shift is made from "cure" to "preparing for death." This change often comes gradually over time. Most of us would like to live as well as possible, as long as possible, even with a bad disease. During the course of the illness we can always prepare for the eventuality of our own death.

Toward the end stages of any disease, more emphasis is placed on the comfort of the patient as opposed to curing the disease. We can come to the point of doing nothing, or very little, to extend the life of the patient. Usually we know the "time is right" when

Most of us would like to live as well as possible, as long as possible, even with a bad disease.

• death is a strong probability;

• available treatments for a fatal condition will likely extend pain and suffering;

• successful treatment is more likely to bring extended unconsciousness or advanced dementia than cure;

• available treatments increase the probability of a death "hooked up to machines" when the patient would have preferred otherwise.[84]

End-Stage Dementia and Comfort Care Only

A patient who does not have decisionmaking capacity and has left no instructions about the appropriate time to refuse curative treatment should be provided reasonable curative care as long as it is not the end-stage of a disease process. When the patient is in the end-stage of dementia, "comfort care only" would appear more appropriate.

Many, if not most, hospice patients have been diagnosed with cancer. **Yet more and more patients at home and in nursing homes suffering from dementia and other "chronic" diseases are entering hospice care or having a "comfort care only" treatment plan.**

Because of the terminal nature of dementia[51] and the clear signs of the approach of the end-stage (see page 25) (although this stage can last for months and even years) many advocate that families consider a "comfort care only" or a hospice treatment plan for these patients.[1,55,56,85-92]

Children and Comfort Care Only

Parents just assume that they will die before their children. I have seen agonizing grief from someone in her 80s who lost a 65-year-old child. It wasn't meant to be this way. And when a child is school-age or younger the unfairness seems more profound.

Yet the harsh reality is that some children do die young. Although none of us would ever want to lose a child, if it were going to happen we would want them to have as peaceful a passing as possible. This takes planning and preparation.[93] The first step toward a comfortable and dignified death is accepting the terminal diagnosis. An earlier recognition of the prognosis contributes to a more peaceful death.[94]

The first step toward a comfortable and dignified death is accepting the terminal diagnosis. An earlier recognition of the prognosis contributes to a more peaceful death.

When can children be involved in medical treatment decisions, especially as it relates to withholding or withdrawing life-sustaining care? They, of course, would have to have the maturity to understand their disease, prognosis, and what treatment options are available to them. Adolescents' opinions probably should be considered.[95] Other children could participate according to their abilities. The American Academy of Pediatrics believes that the views of even younger children should be factored into the end-of-life decisionmaking process.[96]

The emotional and spiritual struggles are the most difficult. It is hard to let go of a child. I once had a 14-year-old patient who lived with his mother. He had a cancer that had filled his chest and arms with tumors. Breathing was so difficult that the most comfortable position for him was to sit on the side of the bed and lean over on a pillow on a tray table. At times, he sat like this day and night. His mother said she wanted everything done to save her son's life including CPR and mechanical ventilators.

One day we talked about her pursuing such aggressive treatment. She was very religious and said, "I figure if I call 911 and he ends up on machines at the hospital, it's God's will. And if I don't call and he dies peacefully here at home, it's God's will." Remembering my principle of "establishing a goal first," I said, "What could you imagine as the most peaceful death your son could have?" She said, "I have thought a lot about that and I just hope one morning I come into his room and find that he died in his sleep." I told her, "The death hooked up to machines is the accident. A peaceful death in his own bed takes planning."

That night, after his father visited, the child relaxed for the first time in days and lay down on the bed. His mother climbed into bed with him. Before long, his breathing stopped. His peaceful death came in his mother's arms. She was able to let go and let be.

Turning From Cure to Comfort Care Only

Patients and families can find great healing when it is time to move away from an emphasis on efforts of curing the disease and moving toward reasonable and more meaningful goals. The alleviation of pain, reconciliation, healing of broken relationships, finding deeper spiritual values, laughing about old times while celebrating the life of the patient, sharing with the patient in the grief and even anger and, of course, saying good-bye are all reasonable hopes for the last days and months of any of our lives. To continue to fight for a cure when there is no reasonable hope for one may cut off the true growth and comfort that can come from going on this journey together with those we love.

Summary:

During the "last phase of life" a time will likely come when the focus shifts from "cure" to "comfort care only" and/or to enter a hospice program.

Hospice is a medical care program designed to keep patients pain-free while paying special attention to the emotional and spiritual needs of both the patient and the family.

Dying in the hospital ICU hooked up to machines and tubes is usually the accident. A peaceful death in one's own bed takes planning.

When advanced dementia reaches the end-stage, it may be appropriate to shift to "comfort care only."

Chapter **Four**

Treatments To Consider—
Practical Help for Decisionmaking

This chapter will answer the following questions:

What are some of the issues one needs to consider when thinking about hospitalization, ventilator support, dialysis, or the use of antibiotics?

How do I communicate my treatment wishes to the medical team caring for me?

What is a "living will" and a "healthcare power of attorney"?

What are some questions that need to be answered to help me make a decision about life-prolonging procedures?

Hospitalization

This is the last of the four most common treatment decisions you might face*. If patients living at home or in a nursing home experience a sudden decline in their health, often they are transferred to a hospital in an effort to restore their health or at least make them more comfortable. Sometimes even patients who want no heroic measures can benefit from such an admission to get symptoms under control or to treat some special need like a possible hip fracture. When considering going into a hospital one must weigh the burdens as well as the possible benefits.

---

*The four most common decisions are: CPR; artificial nutrition and hydration; hospitalization of a nursing home resident or someone living at home; and the hospice approach. (p. 6).

The burdens of hospitalization for the nursing home resident or patient living at home include the following:

- increased possibility of anxiety while getting used to new surroundings, new caregivers, and new routines (this is especially difficult for patients with dementia);[71]
- increased possibility of contracting an infection;
- increased possibility of the use of restraints or sedation, especially for dementia patients;
- increased possibility of aggressively treating any condition because that is the ordinary practice in the hospital; and
- increased possibility of diagnostic testing that may be burdensome or painful and is readily available in the hospital. The testing may be especially burdensome if the patient or family already knows it would not seek treatment for any disease the tests might reveal.

If the resident can receive the same type of care in the nursing home (for example, IV antibiotics), one must ask, why transfer to the hospital? In the rare case when pain can be controlled or comfort assured only in the hospital, hospitalization would be appropriate. Of course, some patients prefer being in the hospital because they feel they get better care. Patient and family preference is a primary concern.

One treatment option to reduce the aggressiveness of medical care is the **"Do Not Hospitalize" order, or DNH.**[97,98] **Some facilities call this "Do Not Transport" to the hospital. This is the essential question, "Can comfort care, pain control, and any desired and appropriate treatment seeking to cure be provided in the nursing home or at home?"** If the answer is "yes," then a DNH order might be considered for the patient. The DNH order is especially helpful if a patient has a change in condition and the attending physician cannot be contacted. The physician on call may have no prior knowledge of the patient's history or of the wishes of the patient or the family in regard to how aggressively to treat the patient. The DNH order helps the physician and staff know about this treatment choice if the family or attending physician cannot be contacted immediately. The DNH order does *not* mean that the patient can *never* be hospitalized but only that the patient will not be hospitalized without a thorough discussion with the patient (if able to make decisions), the family, and the attending physician.[78,79,99-101]

Ventilators

When a person's breathing fails, a machine may be used to aid the patient. This machine is called a ventilator or respirator. Ventilators are commonly used to support respiratory function during and after anesthesia for major operations. Sometimes they may help a patient with severe illnesses such as stroke, pneumonia, or heart failure. When a ventilator is used, the machine is connected to a tube, which is inserted through the mouth and down the windpipe, allowing the machine to force air into the lungs. Sometimes the tube is surgically connected through the throat and directly into the windpipe. This surgical connection is called a "tracheostomy" or "trach."

The tube is uncomfortable and often a patient's hands need to be tied down or the individual is given medication to prevent pulling at the tube, which could dislodge it and cause harm. At times, the medications provide enough comfort so the patient's hands do not need to be tied down. These uncomfortable side effects are acceptable to most people, because the tube and ventilator are removed as soon as the need for them is gone.

But some patients who have a long history of a disease that causes respiratory failure, (like COPD*, emphysema, or heart failure) or neurologic diseases (like Lou Gehrig's disease, ALS**)

*chronic obstructive pulmonary disease   **amyotrophic lateral sclerosis may have to face the possibility that once they are placed on the ventilator they may not be able to get off again. Your physician can help you assess whether or not the use of the ventilator is likely to be temporary or permanent.

For those in respiratory failure there are alternatives to the machine. The physician and the patient could simply use oxygen, a pressurized face mask, a special vest, or medications. As you can imagine, the fear of not being able to breathe can be just as great as the shortness of breath itself. **Medications and supplemental oxygen can be used to address both the fear of being short of breath and the feeling of shortness of breath itself.** I had a patient who had so much difficulty breathing when she moved from the chair to her bed, it took her a half-hour to recover. Yet her chronic shortness of breath was treated very effectively with medication. This conservative elderly lady told me once, "I have always been opposed to drugs. But this morphine is wonderful because it allows me to breathe." Some patients find meditation, prayer, and guided imagery[102] can reduce anxiety, fear, and shortness of breath.

Sometimes patients are put on a ventilator with the hope that its use will be temporary until the pneumonia, heart failure, or other temporary complication is cleared up, but then their health continues to decline with no hope for improvement. The patients or the family may then consider withdrawing the machine, aware that death might be the result. The physician can help you assess what the future might hold. If the decision is made to remove the machine and tube, the patient will be kept comfortable. Pain medications, sedatives, and relaxants will be used as needed to make withdrawal of the artificial respiration comfortable. The family may or may not want to be present. If religious ritual is important to the patient and family, they may want to have clergy present for a prayer before and after the removal of the ventilator. When the ventilator is removed, the person may not die immediately.

Remember, if the patient does die after the withdrawal of a machine, the death is from the disease that caused respiratory failure and **not** from turning off the machine. The patient is not being killed. **By removing the ventilator, we are allowing a natural death to occur that would have happened earlier if the machine had never been started.**[103]

Dialysis

Kidney failure can happen in one of two ways. Persons who have had kidney (renal) decline for a number of years can eventually move into what is known as end-stage renal disease (ESRD). Others may not have had problems before, but in a short time their kidneys fail in what is known as acute renal failure (ARF). Both are very serious conditions, and some patients may be helped with dialysis. In this treatment, blood is circulated from the body of the patient, through a machine that "cleans" the blood of impurities, and pumps it back into the patient. The dialysis process usually does not make people feel better immediately; in fact they often feel wiped out after each treatment. Patients may experience nausea and symptoms of low blood pressure (sweating, dizziness, rapid heart beat, and feeling faint) during the treatments. Patients report a better quality of life on the days they are not dialyzed.

The second most common cause of death for end-stage renal disease . . . is a decision to stop dialysis and die from kidney failure.

For those with acute renal failure, dialysis may keep them alive until their kidneys recover. An ARF dialysis patient who is hospitalized has a 50-75 percent chance of dying during the time in the hospital. For those with end-stage renal disease, the dialysis treatments may keep the patient alive for several years or longer. Patients on dialysis usually die from heart disease or infection. The second most common cause of death for end-stage renal disease, especially patients over the age of 65, is a decision to stop dialysis and die from kidney failure. Approximately one of every five dialysis patients makes a decision to withdraw from dialysis before death.[104] These decisions are usually based on an assessment by the patient that the quality of life is not satisfactory. Without dialysis, ESRD patients usually only live about a week. This is a very peaceful death.

If the patient has one or more other medical problems the risk of death is increased. These risk factors include older age; poor nutritional intake; difficulty or inability to take care of oneself; and diabetes.[105] Your physician and a kidney specialist (nephrologist) can help you assess whether or not dialysis may be an appropriate treatment or is likely to help you. A time-limited trial (see page 27) of the therapy may help the patient learn what the treatment is like and help everyone understand if there is any medical benefit.

If the decision is made to withhold or withdraw dialysis, the patient will be kept comfortable.

If the decision is made to withhold or withdraw dialysis, the medical staff will be able to keep the patient comfortable. Palliative care (comfort care) in the hospital or nursing home and hospice care at home is appropriate for a patient with end-stage renal disease who stops dialysis.

Antibiotics

Before the 1950s, most of the deaths in North America were caused by infections like pneumonia. Antibiotics changed all that, and, fortunately, infections that were once killers often can now be cured. If a person can still swallow, then oral antibiotics pose only a few possible side effects. If an injection or IV is required, then the needle-stick may prove to be minor when compared to the possible benefit. Side effects can include diarrhea, nausea, and vomiting. Throughout most of our lives, antibiotics are routinely taken. But toward the end of life, one might consider not using these medications to allow a natural and peaceful death to occur.

The question of withholding antibiotics usually arises near the end of a long course of a disease like Alzheimer's.[71,106,107] A recurrent problem at the end of Alzheimer's is getting pneumonia because of problems with swallowing. As we have already read (pages 25-26), a feeding tube for such patients is even more likely to cause infection than careful hand feeding. If pneumonia continues to recur after several courses of antibiotics, you may consider not trying them again. Although the medication might temporarily work, it does not cure the underlying problem, the dementia, which continues to progress.

Dying from pneumonia can be very peaceful. **It used to be called "the old person's friend" because of how gently it took someone who had long been disabled by disease.** Your doctor can help you sort through the pros and cons of withholding antibiotics. The physician can also find ways of assuring that the patient will be kept comfortable even though antibiotics are being withheld.

Although I used Alzheimer's as an illustration, not using antibiotics may be a course taken at the end of any disease. I have seen some cancer patients refuse their use. Sometimes the family members of permanently unconscious patients will continue the use of a feeding tube but withhold antibiotics and allow a natural and peaceful death to occur.

Pain Control

Most life-threatening and terminal diseases have pain as a common problem. Fortunately, much can be done to reduce and eliminate any pain. Quite often medications, such as aspirin, acetaminophen (Tylenol), and morphine, are used to alleviate these troublesome symptoms. Other factors besides the disease itself can make pain worse. Depression, spiritual distress, broken family relationships, or lack of sleep can all contribute to increased pain. Likewise, we know that many factors besides drugs can alleviate pain. These are just a few of the things that can contribute to less pain: spiritual counsel from clergy, family, or friends; meditation; music; guided imagery[102]; prayer; hypnosis; visits from family or friends; massage; and many others.

Here are the facts regarding pain control:

- Doctors and/or nurses should ask patients regularly if they are experiencing pain. Never accept pain as inevitable. Always inform your healthcare providers if you are experiencing pain.

- It is important to take pain medications as prescribed. The goal is to stay "ahead of" the pain not just respond when the pain gets unbearable.

- Many patients remain clearheaded while taking pain medications. Others may experience some drowsiness.

- The drowsiness associated with some pain medications usually decreases after several days of taking the medicine.

- Medications used to control pain **DO NOT** become addictive to people who have not had addiction problems in the past.

- Physicians usually increase doses of pain medications like morphine until they find the level needed to control pain. This increasing of dosages is called "titrating." Pain medication that is titrated slowly **WILL NOT** shorten the life of a patient no matter how high the dosage.[108]

- Some patients may choose to be completely sedated (made unconscious by medications) in the last hours or days of life if it is necessary to control pain or other symptoms.[109-115]

Practical Help for Decisionmaking

Treatment decisions are arrived at through an agreement among the physician, the competent patient, and the family. The medical team needs to know what the wishes of the patient are in regard to treatment decisions. There are several things you can do to arrive at a treatment plan and to see that the plan is implemented.

What To Do

1. Discuss the issues. As has already been mentioned, these issues need to be discussed by family members, physicians, and patients who have the mental and emotional capacity for such a discussion. It is best to have such a discussion before a crisis occurs that would require a decision in a time of stress. As with any treatment, you are entitled to a second opinion from another physician.

If you have a difference of opinion with the attending physician, then you have a legal right to transfer the patient's care to another doctor. Likewise, a physician who feels he or she cannot ethically carry out the requests of a family or patient may withdraw from the case.

2. Make an intentional decision.

■ **You want all life-prolonging measures.** After you have discussed the treatment options and decided you would like to have life-prolonging measures applied, usually no special orders are required. These are standard procedures and will most likely be applied if there is no order restricting them. **Delay in making a decision may be interpreted to mean that you want all heroic measures used, including CPR and mechanical ventilators.**

■ **You do not want CPR.** If you do not want CPR used, then ask the physician to write a "do not resuscitate"(DNR), "no CPR" or "no Code" order on the medical record of the patient. If the patient is at home or a nursing home, you may also ask the physician for an "out-of-hospital DNR" form that is honored by the rescue squad (see page 16).

■ **You do not want a feeding tube inserted.** If you do not want a feeding tube inserted, then discuss this with the physician. Generally, you have several days to several weeks to make such a decision if a crisis does occur.

■ **You want artificial feeding withdrawn.** If you want artificial feeding withdrawn, again discuss this with the physician. You must prepare yourself, your family, and your friends emotionally to have such an order carried out. Any of these treatment decisions requires deep emotional involvement, but the decision to withdraw artificial feeding is especially trying.

> *You must prepare yourself emotionally to have artificial feeding withdrawn. . . . this decision is especially trying.*

■ **You do not want to hospitalize a nursing home resident or someone living at home.** If you want to consider a "do not hospitalize" order, contact the attending physician. Explore with the doctor options for keeping the patient comfortable and reaching the medical goals without a transfer to the hospital.

■ **You want a "comfort care only" order or wish to receive palliative care.** Again, this is an order the physician must write, so contact him or her.

■ **You would like to consider participation in a hospice program.** A physician may refer you to a hospice program, or you may contact a local hospice directly through the phone book or contact The National Hospice and Palliative Care Organization (www.caringinfo.org, 800-658-8898).

3. Consider an advance directive. Advance directives generally come in two types: the "living will" or declaration and the Durable Power of Attorney for Health Care. A person must be capable of making decisions in order to establish an advance directive. All states have some form of healthcare advance directive law, which provides for either a living will declaration or a health care proxy, or both.

■ **A living will.** A competent person who does not want to have artificial life-prolonging procedures used when there is no hope of recovery might consider signing a living will. It is called a *living* will because the document takes effect while the person is still living. Typically, the declaration must be signed in the presence of witnesses who are not relatives. Someone holding a power of attorney or a guardian cannot sign the declaration on behalf of another person but they most likely can make decisions for the patient.

The living will states a person's wishes in the event that the person can no longer speak on his or her own behalf.

This declaration states a person's wishes in the event that the person can no longer speak on his or her own behalf. Basically, the declaration says, "If I have a terminal condition, and there is no hope of recovery, I do not want my life prolonged by artificial means." You may add more specific language if you wish or even declare that you *do* want your life artificially prolonged.

Although these laws and declarations are very helpful, some questions still remain. For example, "What is artificial?" As discussed above, some consider feeding tubes "artificial and extraordinary," while others consider them basic medical procedures. Also, "What is terminal?" In one sense, every human is terminal. If a person's heart stops, that is a terminal condition, but for a few patients the condition might be reversed by CPR. If a person cannot eat, that is a terminal condition, although it can be treated by artificial feeding.

In the end, the living will must be interpreted by the family and the physician. They must decide that indeed the ill person is in a "terminal condition, with no hope of recovery" and, therefore, no extraordinary measures will be used. Then they will choose which treatments are extraordinary. Physicians are likely to want to know that *all* the family members agree with a decision to withhold or withdraw treatment even if a living will has clearly stated the patient's desires.[116] A living will is dependent on a family being unified in making sure the patient's wishes are honored. **The realities of these limitations of living wills emphasizes how important it is to have an open, honest, family discussion about treatment choices.**

For more information about advance directives in the United States and a copy of one for your state, go to www.caringinfo.org or call 800-658-8898.

■ **A Durable Power of Attorney for Health Care** (also called a Health Care Proxy) gives the person designated in the document authority to make any healthcare decision on behalf of patients who cannot make decisions for themselves. It covers all healthcare decisions whether or not they relate to terminal illness. The job of the person designated to make decisions is to choose as the patient likely would have decided. Many states now have standard forms to use, or you may want to contact a lawyer for advice regarding this document.

The job of the person designated to make decisions is to choose as the patient likely would have decided.

Questions To Help Make a Decision

1. What is the agreed-upon goal of medical care for the patient at this phase of life? The three possible goals are cure; stabilization of functioning; or preparing for a comfortable and dignified death (see pages 7-10). Remember the goals can be "combined" and will probably change over time, so this and all these questions may need to be revisited from time to time.

2. What does the patient want? Ethicists call this the question of *autonomy*. A patient with decisionmaking capacity who can handle the emotional impact of these questions about life-prolonging procedures can answer without help. If the patient can no longer answer without help, then try to imagine what the patient would have said. To a family who knows the patient's wishes but is hesitant to carry them out, a pastor friend of mine will say, "Sounds like your father has already made up his mind; the question is, are you going to honor it?"

3. What is in the best interest of the patient? This is the question of *values*. You can see from this booklet that there are differences of opinion regarding what is "best" for the patient. Some say it is best to keep a patient alive at all costs. Others say it is best to allow a patient to die and not prolong the dying process with artificial means.

4. What are the prognosis and probable consequences if a certain treatment plan is followed? This is a question to discuss with a physician or an experienced nurse. Other questions related to it are the following: What are the chances of survival after using CPR? If the patient survives, what condition might the patient be in afterwards? Does the physician anticipate just a temporary use of a feeding tube (or other "machines") or might the patient live indefinitely, nonresponsive in a debilitated state? If we try a temporary use of the treatment and the patient does not improve significantly, can the treatment be discontinued? Might death be expected, given the medical condition of the patient? If death would be acceptable and expected, might we try *not* to cure any condition but prepare for a comfortable and dignified death?

5. Can I let go and just let things be? If the answers to the first four questions point to withholding or withdrawing treatment, then this is the most difficult question. Occasionally, a family member will say, "I know my father would never want to be kept alive like this. I know it would be best if he just died. I know there is no hope of his recovery. But I can't let go." Most often, the view of what is medically, ethically, legally, morally, or according to my religion, appropriate treatment, is totally influenced by the question, "Can I let go and let be?" This is discussed more thoroughly in the next chapter.

Getting Help with End-of-Life Decisions

Are decisions regarding life-prolonging procedures black and white? No! They are often shades of gray. As you gather more information, the answers will become clearer. Physicians, nurses, clergy, and social workers are just a few of the people who can help you sort out the decision. **The medical staff caring for the patient will be as supportive as possible, no matter what the treatment decision.**

Summary:

As a patient's condition declines you may be faced with decisions about hospitalization, ventilator support, dialysis, or even the use of antibiotics. For some patients these treatments are appropriate and for others they may be withheld.

Written "living wills" and "durable powers of attorney for health care" can be helpful, but the most important thing one can do for future care is to discuss your wishes with your family and physician.

In making decisions about life-prolonging procedures, first establish the goal of the treatment then consider what the patient wants, what's in the best interest of the patient, and what the prognosis is.

If most of the signs seem to be pointing toward withholding or withdrawing treatment, the big question is "Can I let go and let be?"

Chapter *Five*

The Journey to Letting Be

This chapter will answer the following questions:
What is the author's personal opinion about
these treatments?
Is it possible to let go and let be?
Are there others who have experienced this "letting go
and letting be" who can show the way?

Since 1983, I have served as a chaplain in a nursing home, a hospice program and a hospital. My convictions on life-prolonging procedures have grown out of my pastoral relationship with patients and their families. My teachers have been the patients, their families, caring nurses, physicians, medical research, and writings reflecting on the emotional and spiritual struggles at the end of life.

A Personal Word From a Chaplain–
The Four Treatment Decisions

Here is where I am today on each of the four most common treatment decisions for patients toward the end of their lives. Although I believe my opinions have a solid foundation in research and my own experience, nothing can substitute for a discussion of these issues with your physician, family, and spiritual guides.

1. **CPR.** I recognize that 15 percent of hospital patients do survive after CPR.[5] A physician can help the patient and

the family assess if resuscitation attempts offer any possible medical benefit.

The evidence overwhelmingly shows that CPR is not able to restore most patients who are at the end of a life-threatening illness to their previous level of functioning. CPR is of no medical benefit to these patients. In two studies, almost all the nursing home patients who are successfully resuscitated and discharged from the hospital refuse any further CPR attempts.[7,14,117] I think this speaks about their own or their family's assessment of the benefit of CPR.

One researcher referred to the practice of discussing CPR with failing patients at the end of their lives or their families as a "cruel hoax." The hoax is that we approach those making medical decisions for the patient and ask whether or not to use CPR, which implies that it offers some benefit.[16,118] In its most cruel form, this is like asking, "Do you want us to attempt CPR or do you want us to let your mother die?"

Refusing resuscitation attempts is not giving up hope on life.

Who *wants* their mother to die? The fact is, that is the wrong question. These patients are going to die with or without CPR. For various reasons (some of them very good), the system in this country requires us to ask permission *not* to do a treatment that has been proven not only to be ineffective but even harmful to certain patients. Therefore, we make patients and families feel they are making the *choice* to let someone die. **The real choice is whether the patient will die a more peaceful death or one spent in its final moments with all the force of our medical aggressiveness attempting to reverse certain death.**

My observation has been that families who want their dying relatives to receive CPR are having a difficult time letting go and letting be. They have watched the slow decline of a once-vital person. For them to say "do not use CPR" is like saying "I give up hope." **But refusing resuscitation attempts is not giving up hope on life. It is facing the fact that there is no hope that CPR will save the life of this patient.** CPR becomes merely a symbol, meaning, "We never gave up trying." Since it offers no medical benefit, it is a meaningless symbol. A genuine question a family must ask is, "Are we wanting Mother to receive CPR for us or for her? Is it because we cannot accept the fact that she is going to die some day that we want everything done to keep her alive?" **Most often the loving thing to do is to let her die in peace without the aggressiveness of CPR.**

2. Artificial Hydration and Nutrition. The question of artificial hydration and nutrition is not quite as clear for me. Perhaps the best friend I made at the nursing home was a 42-year-old Navy Commander who had ALS (Lou Gehrig's disease). He could talk with difficulty, or if talking did not work, he would use his toe to draw letters in order to spell out words. We would discuss world events, tell jokes, and share stories about our families. His life was sustained by a mechanical respirator and by an artificial feeding tube. He found a way to make the best of his situation. Given the same handicaps, I hope I would choose to go on with life as he did. Fortunately, he was competent and could make his own choice to be "kept alive" through artificial means.

I have seen other patients have a tube inserted as a temporary measure for hydration and nutrition. After they regained their strength, the tube was removed and they returned to swallowing normally.

On the other hand, many patients who have no hope of regaining their ability to eat or drink are sustained through artificial feeding. Some seem to respond with their eyes as if trying to speak. Others make no purposeful response, no eye contact, and no sounds to indicate they are trying to talk.

I have often been at the bedsides of people who have lived for years in a nonresponsive condition.

The permanent inability to take in food or water is a terminal condition. **As with any terminal condition, one has the right to refuse artificial feeding, just as one has the right to refuse CPR or a respirator.**

The permanent inability to take in food or water is a terminal condition.

I have been involved in more than a dozen cases where artificial feeding was begun and later stopped, allowing the person to die.

One case involved an 83-year-old woman who suffered a stroke and had a feeding tube inserted. She never again made any sort of appropriate response to her environment. Two and a half years after the stroke, her leg broke when the nurses routinely turned her. Her three sons were convinced she would never have wanted to be sustained like that and asked the doctor to withdraw the artificial feeding and let her die.

A 40-year-old woman had a brain tumor and through a series of events ended up in a persistent vegetative state after undergoing an operation. She received feeding through a tube for more than 2 years. The patient's physician told the family, "If this were my daughter, I would stop the feedings and let her die." The family agreed and took her home to spend her last days. Years after the patient's death, I was visiting with her mother. She said, "You helped me so much as we were struggling with our decision. Remember the day I came into your office crying, worried that I would be killing my daughter if we stopped the feedings?" I told her I remembered it well. She went on, "You told me I wasn't killing her but the brain tumor was."

Another woman had been at the nursing home for about 5 years and had had two strokes. She was able to sit in a wheelchair, eat and visit with her family, but she was not satisfied with her quality of life. She had a third stroke, which the family had expected some day. Rather than rush her to the hospital, where she would likely have received a feeding tube, and knowing their mother's wishes, the family and physician decided to keep her at the nursing home. She could not take in any food or fluid by mouth. She was alert, and her eyes seemed to follow people as they moved around the room. We kept her comfortable and free from pain. She died peacefully a week later. This family made the courageous decision not to start a feeding tube that would only prolong the dying process, perhaps for years.

Ideally people should make an intentional choice either to accept or refuse artificial feedings. My observations have led me to believe that often people will receive feeding tubes without the doctors' allowing families or patients to make a choice. I am sure physicians are afraid of the legal ramifications of "not trying everything." I wish doctors would offer a time-limited trial of a feeding tube (see page 27). If it does not have the desired effect in the specified time, then a choice could be made to continue or discontinue. But people

Curiously, many cultures see stopping eating as a sign of dying and not its cause. They never even consider the use of a feeding tube.

get into a situation where they had hoped a tube would be temporary, and years later the patient has still not made any sort of response.

Some families do make a conscious choice to continue tube feedings even when there is no response from the patient. The daughter of one such patient told me, "I could never not feed Mother." I respected her position. If she let her mother die, she, not I, would have to live with that decision. I know she was sure she would feel guilty if she approved of the withdrawal of treatment and let her mother die. In the whole of human history, it is only in this generation (and mostly in the United States[60]) that families feel guilty if they do not artificially feed someone who stops eating at the end of life.

Curiously, many cultures see stopping eating as a *sign* of dying and not its *cause*. They never even consider the use of a feeding tube. We humans stop taking in food and fluid as part of our systems shutting down. It was like we were created to go out of this world as gently as possible and the way we have done this since the beginning of time is to stop eating and drinking at the end of life. Yet, now, some would say we are "starving a patient to death" if we do not artificially force feed them.[119,120]

Like the patients in a permanently unconscious state, I believe that artificial feeding of those with end-stage Alzheimer's disease or other dementias is a totally inappropriate treatment. It does not cure the underlying disease, it does not prevent death, and it does not even offer a longer life than for those who do not receive a tube. The numerous burdens of a feeding tube for these patients are not counterbalanced by any benefit (see pages 25-26).

As in the case of CPR, treatment has become symbolic.[121] All cultures through all ages offer food and water as a sign of hospitality and caring. But when a patient can no longer receive sustenance by mouth, artificially supplied feeding no longer carries the same meaning for me. Artificially fed patients receive little of the emotional and spiritual support a patient may receive through hand feeding, although they obviously can be loved and cared for in other ways. But artificial feeding for terminally ill, dying, or otherwise failing patients becomes only a symbol for the family and has little medical benefit for the patient.

I have seen a more powerful symbol of caring than using a feeding tube. In my early years as a nursing home chaplain a woman came to us from the hospital with a feeding tube that she had received after a stroke. After she repeatedly pulled it out, her daughter, a nurse, and I went in to speak with the patient. She clearly understood she would die without the tube and that was her wish. The daughter accepted her mother's decision. I will never forget the last time I saw them. I rounded the corner to enter the mother's room, only to see that her daughter had climbed into bed with the patient. The younger woman cradled her elderly mother in her arms. They were silent. Words were not required. Which is a more powerful symbol of love and caring? A daughter cuddling her mother in her last days or artificially supplied feeding? In my dying, I would wish for the loving touch.

> *"The ultimate tragedy is depersonalization . . . dying in an alien and sterile arena, separated from the spiritual nourishment that comes from being able to reach out to a loving hand."*
>
> Norman Cousins

I am reminded of Norman Cousins' words, "Death… is not the ultimate tragedy. The ultimate tragedy is depersonalization… dying in an alien and sterile arena, separated from the spiritual nourishment that comes from being able to reach out to a loving hand."[122]

3. Hospitalization. I have seen very effective use of a decision not to treat a nursing home resident or person living at home in the hospital. By design, hospitals are more aggressive in the treatment of diseases. When patients are in declining health and have an acute illness, it often seems appropriate to provide care only in the nursing home or at home.

Sometimes hospitalization seems to be the only choice for something like a possible hip fracture. I have been amazed at the recovery of some very elderly residents from a hip replacement. On the other hand, sometimes hospitalization for such surgery is the beginning of the end. I have no real sense of how to know ahead of time into which category a patient would fall. We do know that half of all end-stage dementia patients who are hospitalized for a hip fracture or pneumonia will die within six months as compared to 12-13 percent of mentally intact patients.[56] Families and patients must confer with physicians and nurses as to what is appropriate for *this* patient at *this* time. As a general rule, hospitalization should be reserved for patients who cannot have their comfort needs or treatment goals met at the nursing home or in their own home, but might have these needs met in the hospital.

4. Hospice and the "Comfort Care Only" Order. Hospice is most effective when a patient and family enter a program months before the patient actually dies. An earlier shifting to a "comfort care only" order for nursing home or home-bound patients is also ideal. Sadly, some people put off shifting the focus from attempts to cure to improving quality of life until the very end stage of the disease process. These patients and families miss the full benefit of hospice and the "comfort care only" order.

Sadly, some people put off shifting the focus from attempts to cure to improving quality of life until the very end stage of the disease process. These patients and families miss the full benefit of hospice and the "comfort care only" order.

The beauty of this approach is that the family, patient, and medical team are no longer being consumed with aggressive attempts to achieve a cure. All physical symptoms continue to be addressed, but the emphasis shifts to the alleviation of pain and to giving emotional and spiritual care to the dying person and the family. With cure no longer being the primary goal, the patient and family are able to do the difficult but more important work of improving the patient's quality of life, saying good-bye, grieving together, and sharing in one of the most important events in the life of the family.

Changing the Treatment Plan

One of my goals in writing this booklet was to introduce those who are making medical care decisions for a patient to the wide range of what is acceptable from legal, ethical, moral, and medical points of view. What makes the difference in choosing one treatment plan over another?

In my years of experience as a healthcare chaplain, I have thought much about medical interventions on behalf of patients at the end of their lives. I have considered CPR, artificial feeding, IV therapy on the dying patient, hospitalization, and even the use of antibiotics and diagnostic work on failing patients. Often, in the eyes of my colleagues on the medical team and in my own opinion, these treatments are not medically indicated, marginal in their benefit (if there is any benefit at all), increase the burden of living, possibly prolong the dying process, and are not required by ethics, medicine, law, morality, or faith. Why are they done?

Perhaps the reason these treatments are pursued is that the family has not been able to let go (and the physician has also not been able to let go or has not informed the decisionmakers of the marginal benefit of such treatment plans). **Those who choose such life-prolonging treatments for failing patients do so primarily out of an inability to let go and not out of moral necessity or medical appropriateness.**[123,124] How else can you explain such a wide range of treatment choices for similarly afflicted patients?

I see these emotional and spiritual struggles often overwhelming all other considerations. Caregivers who share cultural and religious backgrounds will still choose different treatment plans because one caregiver is having a harder time letting go.[7,125-128] This is especially obvious when brothers and sisters choose different treatments. I have many times heard, "The rest of us had made the decision to let Mom go, but our brother wasn't ready yet." Another reason I know that decisions are mostly based on the emotional and spiritual struggle of letting go is because I have seen so many family members change from an aggressive treatment plan to withdrawal of

Words to Try
For Families, Talking with a Sick Person

When you think you want to say:	Try this instead:
Dad, you are going to be just fine.	Dad, are there some things you worry about?
Don't talk like that! You can beat this!	It must be hard to come to terms with all this.
I can't see how anyone can help.	We will be there for you, always.
I just can't talk about this.	I am feeling a little overwhelmed right now. Can we take this up later tonight?
What do the doctors know? You might live forever.	Do you think the doctors are right? How does it seem to you?
Please don't give up. I need you here.	I need you here. I will miss you terribly. But we will get through somehow.
There has to be something more to do.	Let's be sure we get the best of medical treatments, but let's be together when we have done all we can.
Don't be glum. You will get well.	It must be hard. Can I just sit with you for a while?

From *Handbook for Mortals: Guidance for People Facing Serious Illness*, p. 11, by Joanne Lynn and Joan Harrold, Copyright © 1999 by Joanne Lynn. Used by permission of Oxford University Press, Inc.

62

curative treatment. **Decisionmakers do not usually have a change of *mind* about ethics, law, morality, or religion. They have a change of *heart*. They finally come to the point of being able to let go and just let things be.**

The Emotional Nature of the Struggle–Treating the Wrong Patient

A friend came to me on a Monday and was fighting back tears when she said, "I have to make a life-and-death decision about my mother by Thursday." My friend was about a 3-hour drive from the town where her mother was hospitalized. Her 82-year-old mother's health had been failing for 2 years. In that time she had had two strokes, was in kidney failure, and at the time was in the hospital on dialysis. My friend and her family were facing the decision of whether or not to withdraw the dialysis.

Thinking of the questions to help make a decision, I asked, "How effectively is the dialysis working?"

"Oh. The doctors say it isn't doing any good."

I asked, "Did your mother ever give any indication of what she would have wanted?"

"Yes. She said she never wanted to be on dialysis."

I couldn't believe what I was hearing. I said, "I am going to be straight with you because you are a friend. This is not a hard decision. There is no question that you stop treatment. What is going on here that makes this so difficult?"

She began to choke up again, fighting back tears, "I guess I am feeling guilty for not having visited my mother enough these last couple of years." At least she was honest enough with herself to know the real issue. A patient was being treated miles away in order to take care of a daughter's guilt. This happens more often than we would like to admit.

Once a physician wrote an order to start an IV to hydrate a dying patient, and he said to the nurse, "We're doing this for the family." He knew that this treatment probably would not add to the patient's comfort and might even contribute to her discomfort. But he was doing *something* for an emotionally distraught family. I wish he had said to the family, "I know you are struggling with the fact that your mother is dying. None of us wants to lose our mother. But starting an IV will not help her nor stop her eventual death. But I am concerned about you and want the nurse to call the chaplain or social worker so you can talk about what you are struggling with. We will keep your mother comfortable and as free from pain as possible."

Sometimes it seems easier to aggressively treat patients, perhaps even for years, than to help families confront the emotional and spiritual issues that are driving the treatment choices. Indeed, physicians are trained to order medical treatments and not necessarily to help patients and families with the more difficult struggles in their souls. It is understandable that they would address a family's emotional struggle by ordering aggressive treatment of a patient. The problem is, they are treating the wrong patient.

> *Can you let go and let be? Of course you can. . . . And it can take a long or a short time.*

Can I Let Go and Let Be?

Once a daughter told me, as her father was very close to death, "I know a 'no CPR' order is the best thing, but I just can't let go." She wasn't talking about medical or even ethical decisions. She was in the midst of an emotional struggle to let go. Her holding on was just an illusion. Perhaps she felt CPR attempts would allow her to hold on to her father for just a little longer, but in actuality that treatment could not accomplish that goal. She finally requested the "no CPR" order only days before his death.

We had another patient in his 80s fed by an artificial feeding tube. In 4 years at the nursing home, he rarely made any response to those around him. His wife could answer the questions I asked to help her make a decision whether or not to withdraw the artificial feeding and let her husband die. She said, "I know he would never have wanted to be kept alive like this. I know it would be best if he just died. I know he will never get better. But I just can't let go."

She struggled with the withdrawal of treatment decision for more than 2 years. It finally came down to a meeting with an administrator, a daughter, the wife, her pastor and me. We reviewed the patient's condition and what his wishes would have been. The minister asked if the administrator and I would leave the room for a minute. When he called us back in, the wife said she had decided to withdraw the treatment and let her husband die. She signed a document authorizing the withdrawal of the artificial feeding. I will never forget her next words, "I feel like a great burden has been lifted from my shoulders." She had let go and let be.

Can you let go and let be? Of course you can, though some people never do. And it can take a long or a short time. As a pastoral caregiver, I wonder how I can help families and patients come to the place of letting go and letting be. Years after the event, I even called three family members of two patients who died after the withdrawal of artificial feeding. I asked each, "Did you have any regrets in your decision to withdraw treatment?" Without knowing what the others had said, they each immediately responded, "Yes. I regret that we did not withdraw treatment sooner." Then I asked, "Was there anything either I or the nursing center could have done to help you come to this decision sooner?" Again, they all responded, "No. It just takes time."

It is because of this element of time that I have seen the families of dementia patients tend to more readily accept

letting go of the patient in the end.[55,129] Because of the slow progression of the disease, the family has been having to let go of parts of this person for years. They have already been grieving and letting go, and therefore they find saying "no CPR" or no artificial feeding tube is the next step in releasing this person. I do not mean to imply that this decision is "easy" for anyone. Yet, because of the emotional nature of these decisions, families of patients with dementia have already been going through much of this letting go and letting be.

A Lifetime of Letting Go

After describing the difficult and sometimes painful struggles people go through in letting go of someone at the end of life, a massage therapist friend of mine said, "This is the same issue my clients are dealing with. They come with a stiff neck or back pain. They have to learn how to let go."

I do not mean to imply that this decision is "easy" for anyone. Yet, because of the emotional nature of these decisions, families of patients with dementia have already been going through much of this letting go and letting be.

A natural response to the possibility of losing someone is to hold on tighter or to try to gain more control. Ironically, this does not lead to a life of freedom and joy, the very things we were pursuing. Most of us do learn to let go. We let go of our childhood and accept adult responsibilities. We let go of our teenage children and our attempts to control them. We let go of finding happiness in possessions or careers. We even learn that we have to let go of other people and not be dependent on them for our happiness. To learn these lessons, we have to accept the fact that these things or people were gifts in the first place.

There are two ways to hold on. We can grasp tightly as we would a coin in our fist. We fear we will lose it, so we hold it tight. Indeed, if we open our hand palm down the coin falls from our possession, and we feel cheated. The other way to hold on is by opening our hand palm up. The coin may sit there, or it could be blown away or shaken out of our "possession." But while it is there, we are privileged to have it. We hold on with an open hand. Our hand is relaxed and we experience freedom.[130]

I do not want to trivialize or oversimplify the deep struggles within our hearts as we make end-of-life decisions. **Yet I am convinced that letting go and letting be is a way of life that can be experienced throughout our lifetime.** Grasping, controlling individuals tend to be so to the very end of life. Those who live life with a sense of gift and grace also tend to do so to the very end of life.[131] Daniel Callahan writes,

> How we die will be an expression of how we have wanted to live, and the meaning we find in our dying is likely to be at one with the meaning we have found in our living.... [A] person who has learned how to let life go may have not only a richer and more flexible life, but also one that better prepares him for his decline.[132]

Throughout most of our lives, aggressive curative medical treatment is appropriate. Those who live life with a sense of grace and letting go can seek a cure from diseases from which they would have a reasonable opportunity to recover. But those who have a sense of giftedness of life have an easier time letting go when treatment has a limited possibility of cure and a greater possibility of increasing burden.

Two studies uncovered the fact that CPR is used less in religious nursing homes.[6,7] It was not the purpose of these studies to find out why there is less CPR in these religious homes, but one reason may be because they have a positive view of life after death. I do not feel that adequately explains the difference in the use of CPR. My guess is that the administration and staff have a sense that life is a gift and to hold on too tightly is to betray the sense of giftedness. They live daily with an open hand, appreciating each moment and not having to control events—including not having to stop death. By their presence, they then communicate this lifestyle to patients and families. I hope my faith is a faith for living fully each day with a sense of grace and gift. Then when I can no longer have this gift of life, I do not have to grasp it either for myself or for those I love.

When I can no longer have this gift of life, I do not have to grasp it either for myself or for those I love.

Some Religious Questions

Sometimes a family member, choosing aggressive life-prolonging treatment like CPR or a mechanical ventilator, says something like, "When God calls a person home, then they will go, no matter what we do." The patient then continues to be kept alive on the machine. But I believe some things we do *can* stop people from being "called home."

What greater message could a body be giving us that it is "time to go" than the heart stopping? When a body can no longer take in food in the natural way, we might be "playing God" by inserting a feeding tube. Then again, we might be playing God by not using all the technology "He has given us." There are no easy answers.

I would rather not make assumptions about what God is trying to tell us through someone's medical condition. Not that we should approach these decisions without prayer and the counsel of our spiritual guides. But we cannot presume that God is trying to tell us something one way or the other.

Just because we have been "blessed" with certain technology does not mean we are obliged to use it.

On my first visit into the home of a woman with advanced metastatic cancer the husband said, "Hank, God has told me that my wife is not going to die so I don't want any negative talk about death and dying, only positive thoughts of healing." I said I would honor that but that I usually let the patient and family set the agenda and if the topic of dying came up I would discuss it.

I believe we are on dangerous ground thinking we get a clear divine message that someone with advanced end-stage cancer will not die when the death expectancy rate for all of us is 100 percent.

A month or so later they had gotten the news that the cancer had spread to yet another organ. When I arrived for a visit the husband was preparing to go out the door to work. "You know how I told you, God has told me my wife is going to live?" he started. "Well, I still believe that but Satan is trying to get me to doubt it. Would you pray for me?" I said of course I would. He left and I turned to his wife and asked her if she had as much confidence that she would not die as her husband did. She said no and began to cry. Through her tears she said, "I am afraid if I die I will be disappointing my husband."

On my next visit I told him what she had said. He sat close to her, took her hand, and assured her that she could never disappoint him. I said I had two concerns about only talking of healing in the midst of such a grave condition. "My first is that you may not adequately control the pain under the logic that since she is not dying let's just give her Tylenol." I continued, "My other concern is that you will miss having some very important conversations if you do not allow for the possibility of death. We all need to live as if each day were our last but in your situation, having that attitude is most important."

After her death he said that he knew that God told him "she will not die" because God felt he wouldn't be able to handle the truth. I don't like to speak for God but I just do not believe that the Lord intentionally tells us a lie. In my opinion, this man so much wanted to hear the words "your wife will not die" that he imagined it came from God. It is perfectly understandable for him to not want to lose his wife. And it is surely appropriate to pray for healing. But I believe we are on dangerous ground thinking we get a clear divine message that someone with advanced end-stage cancer will not die when the death expectancy rate for all of us is 100 percent.

The Spiritual Nature of the Struggle

Although a few may have these questions about God or religion, we all ask the deeper spiritual questions as we contemplate the end of life. When I say "spiritual," try not to think of religion, a place of worship, or an organized way of thinking about God. I am using the word in the broader sense of "that which gives life ultimate meaning." Spiritual, in this sense, denotes that essence of ourselves that is greater than the flesh and bones that we inhabit. We are confronted most profoundly with our spiritual nature when someone we love is dying or does die. After the breath of life has gone out and the blood no longer gives vitality to the flesh, what is the meaning of this person's life?

Sadly, most people spend much of their life avoiding this ultimate question.[133-135] We surround ourselves with things and activities to mask the reality of the truth of our impermanence. We grasp on to life and our loved ones who are on the edge of dying. But the grasping can bring as much spiritual pain as the dying itself. Many times I sat in our hospice team meeting as we discussed a family who was struggling so hard to hold on. They were grasping and controlling. I have said, "Dying is hard enough as it is. These people are making it so much harder than it needs to be." Sogyal Rinpoche writes,

> *"God, grant me the serenity to accept the things I cannot change; the courage to change the things I can; and the wisdom to know the difference."*[145]
>
> Reinhold Niebuhr

We are terrified of letting go, terrified, in fact, of living at all, since learning to live is learning to let go. And this is the tragedy and the irony of our struggle to hold on: not only is it impossible, but it brings us the very pain we are seeking to avoid.[136]

This teaching of the impermanence of life can be found in all cultures, religions, and ages. The Psalmist wrote, "For he knows how we were made; he remembers that we are dust. As for mortals, their days are like grass; they flourish like a flower of the field; for the wind passes over it, and it is gone, and its place knows it no more."[137] Yet it seems in our current culture, we make every effort to deny its existence and fight "to the very end," to say "it ain't so." **It is at this point—whether or not we accept the certainty of our own death and the deaths of those we love—where making end-of-life decisions becomes, at bottom, a spiritual issue.** To let go, we must have the sense that this person will be okay even in death.

Giving Up, Letting Go, and Letting Be

A psychotherapist told me a man who was struggling with AIDS once said, "I have finally learned the difference between giving up and letting go." I have reflected often on his thoughts and see them as a struggle we all go through. This is especially true as we wrestle with end-of-life decisions.

The truth is that we will die whether we give up, let go, or let be. We are making a choice about the nature of our dying or the dying of one we love. **We die in trust and grace or in fear and struggle.** Perhaps I titled my booklet improperly. We are not faced with many hard choices. We are faced with one hard choice. **Can we let go and live life out of grace or must we hold on out of fear? Or can we just let things be?**

That is really what we are talking about, "letting things be." To withhold or withdraw artificial and mechanical devices is just returning the patient to a natural state. We are

Giving Up, Letting Go, and Letting Be

Giving up implies a struggle
  Letting go implies a partnership
    Letting be implies, in reality, there is nothing that
      separates

Giving up says there is something to lose
  Letting go says there is something to gain
    Letting be says it doesn't matter

Giving up dreads the future
  Letting go looks forward to the future
    Letting be accepts the present as the only moment I
      ever have

Giving up lives out of fear
  Letting go lives out of grace and trust
    Letting be just lives

Giving up is defeat at the hands of suffering
  Letting go is victory over suffering
    Letting be knows suffering is often in my own mind in
      the first place

Giving up is unwillingly yielding control to forces beyond myself
  Letting go is choosing to yield to forces beyond myself
    Letting be acknowledges that control and choices can
      be illusions

Giving up believes that God is to be feared
  Letting go trusts in God to care for me
    Letting be never asks the question

Hank Dunn

accepting what is. We have come to accept that the patient is dying and we will just let be.[138]

Viktor Frankl was a psychiatrist and a Jew who was imprisoned for several years in Nazi concentration camps. As he observed the behavior of the inmates, of the guards, and of himself, he asked the question, "Can life have meaning in such horrible conditions?" His answer was "yes." I refer to those who suffered under the Nazis, not to make light of their suffering. Indeed, their suffering had an element of evil that none of us hope to ever have to face. That is my point. If they, in such awful circumstances, can find hope and meaning, surely I can in whatever hardships life brings my way.

Of the many stories Frankl relates, I have been most moved by the reflections of a young woman as she lay dying. In this story is the essence of letting go and letting be and the assurance that, at bottom, the universe is a caring place:

> This young woman knew that she would die in the next few days. But when I talked to her she was cheerful in spite of this knowledge. "I am grateful that fate has hit me so hard," she told me. "In my former life I was spoiled and did not take spiritual accomplishments seriously." Pointing through the window of the hut, she said, "This tree here is the only friend I have in my loneliness." Through that window she could see just one branch of a chestnut tree, and on the branch were two blossoms. "I often talk to this tree," she said to me. I was startled and didn't quite know how to take her words. Was she delirious? Did she have occasional hallucinations? Anxiously I asked her if the tree replied. "Yes." What did it say to her? She answered, "It said to me, 'I am here—I am here—I am life, eternal life.'"[139]

If a woman dying in a concentration camp can see that there is goodness, that there is life, then what is wrong with my vision?

Fatal Isn't the Worst Outcome

Often we gain the greatest insights on how to live from those closest to death. Many who have a near-death experience in which they were considered dead and are brought back to life report that the "other side" is a wonderful place and their fear of death is gone.[140-142] Their lives are changed for the better after that experience.

Sandol Stoddard reports conversations with hospice patients:

> "Let me tell you, Doctor," said an eighty-three-year-old Hospice of Marin patient, "dying is the experience of a lifetime." What she meant by these splendid words remains, like the fabric of life itself, a mystery. "I think I was meant to come here," says Lillian Preston's final letter from St. Christopher's Hospice, "so that at last, I could experience joy." "I never knew how to live until I came here to die," said an elderly, blind gentleman of St. Joseph's Hospice in London.[143]

It sounds paradoxical: by excluding death from our life we cannot live a full life, and by admitting death into our life we enlarge and enrich it.

Etty Hillesum

Certainly families, friends and the larger community are saddened and grieve the loss of someone we love. Yet we still have to incorporate this loss into our larger understanding of the meaning of life. Etty Hillesum, who would eventually die in the Auschwitz concentration camp, wrote about her contemplation of her own death. She said,

> "The reality of death has become a definite part of my life; my life has, so to speak, been extended by death, by my looking death in the eye and accepting it, by accepting destruction as part of life and no longer wasting my energies on fear of death or the refusal to acknowledge its inevitability. It sounds paradoxical: by excluding death from our life we cannot live a full life, and by admitting death into our life we enlarge and enrich it."[144]

My wish is that patients with serious and life-threatening illnesses, their families, and physicians would have the grace to accept that a time comes when certain medical treatments only prolong the dying process. May they also have the wisdom to know when that time comes. And in those moments of letting go and letting be may they have a sense of being upheld by a loving God in the midst of a caring universe.

Philosophers, sages, and saints through the ages often show a profound appreciation that the essence of life is to live each day fully and that a life is not negated by death. My hope is that patients and families will concentrate on living each day fully while accepting modern medicine's inability to extend the length of life indefinitely.

As conservationist Edward Abbey thought about the ending of his short 62 years, he commented, "It is not death or dying which is tragic, but rather to have existed without fully participating in life is the deepest personal tragedy."[147] Dr. Bernie Siegel works with people who are living with cancer. He has formed groups for patients called ECaP groups, for Exceptional Cancer Patients. A group member said one day, "Fatal isn't the worst outcome." And Siegel adds, "Not living is the worst outcome."[148]

My message to those who are taking this journey to letting go and letting be is one of hope. We can live each day fully even as we accept the certainty of our own death and that of those we love. To accept medicine's inability to put off death indefinitely is not a defeat. On the one hand, it is accepting the world as it was created, while at the same time having a profound sense that the Creator has granted life as a gift. For me to hold on and grasp out of fear is to deny the gift and the Giver. Having walked this journey to letting be with hundreds of patients and families, I only have a greater sense of the wonderfulness of life.

Hank Dunn, Chaplain

Endnotes
See **www.hardchoices.com** for links to endnotes.

Abbreviations: *BMJ = British Medical Journal; JAGS=Journal of the American Geriatrics Society; AJHPM= American Journal of Hospice and Palliative Medicine; JAMA = Journal of the American Medical Association; NEJM = New England Journal of Medicine*

1. Lynn J. Dying and dementia (editorial). *JAMA* 1986;256:2244-45.
2. Youngner S. Healthcare Challenges of Medically Futile Care. Issues in Medical Ethics , Medical University of South Carolina, 1994.
3. Kaldjian LC et al. Goals of care toward the end of life: A structured literature review. *AJHPM* 2009;25:501-11.
4. National Conference for Cardiopulmonary Resuscitation (CPR) and Emergency Cardiac Care (ECC): Standards for CPR and ECC. *JAMA* 1974;227:864-6.
5. Saklayen M, Liss H, Markert R. In-hospital cardiopulmonary resuscitation: Survival in 1 hospital and literature review. *Medicine* 1995;74:163-75. Patients with the greatest chance of survival: those who experience a certain kind of abnormal heart rhythm (ventricular tachycardia or fibrillation) (21 percent survived); those with respiratory arrest only; and those who were generally healthy and the cardiac or respiratory arrest was their only medical problem.
6. Duthie E et al. Utilization of CPR in nursing homes in one community: Rates and nursing home characteristics. JAGS 1993;41:384-8.
7. Finucane TE et al. The incidence of attempted CPR in nursing homes. *JAGS* 1991;39:624-6.
8. Varon J, Marik PE. Cardiopulmonary resuscitation in patients with cancer. *AJHPM* 2007;24(3):224-9.
9. Peberdy MA et al. Cardiopulmonary resuscitation of adults in the hospital: A report of 14,720 cardiac arrests from the National Registry of Cardiopulmonary Resuscitation. *Resuscitation* 2003;58:297-308.
10. Booth CM et al. Is this patient dead, vegetative, or severely neurologically impaired? Assessing outcome for comatose survivors of cardiac arrest. *JAMA* 2004;291:870-79.
11. Ebell M et al. Survival after in-hospital cardiopulmonary resuscitation: A meta-analysis. *J of General Internal Med* 2001;13(12):805-16.
12. Terminal disease is "advanced, irreparable organ failures (decompensated cirrhosis of the liver, uremia not amenable to dialysis, New York Heart Association Stage IV congestive heart failure, advanced metastatic cancer, sepsis, anoxic encephalopathy, irreversible respiratory failure)." Saklayen M see note 5 above.
13. Applebaum GE, King JE, Finucane TE. The outcome of CPR initiated in nursing homes. *JAGS* 1990;38:197-200.
14. Tresch DD et al. Outcomes of cardiopulmonary resuscitation in nursing homes: Can we predict who will benefit? *Am J Med* 1993;95:123-30.
15. Awoke S, Mouton CP, Parrott M. Outcomes of skilled CPR in a long-term-care facility: Futile therapy? *JAGS* 1992;40:593-5.
16. Gordon M et al. Poor outcome of on-site CPR in a multi-level geriatric facility: 3 1/2 years experience at the Baycrest Centre for Geriatric Care. *JAGS* 1993;41:163-6.
17. McIntyre KM. Failure of 'predictors' of CPR outcomes to predict CPR outcomes (editorial). *Arch Intern Med* 1993;153:1293-6.
18. Colburn D. The 40-year vigil for Rita Greene. *The Washington Post* Health Section,10-13, Mar 12, 1991 and Obituaries, *The Washington Post* B6, Feb 3, 1999.
19. Maslow K. Total parenteral nutrition and tube feeding for elderly patients: Findings of an OTA study. *Parenter Enteral Nutr* 1988;12:425-32.
20. Cranford RE. The persistent vegetative state: The medical reality (getting the facts straight) *Hastings Center Report* Feb/Mar 1988:27-32.
21. Zerwekh J. Do dying patients really need IV fluids? *Am J Nurs* 1997:26-30.
22. Ellershaw JE, Sutcliffe JM, Saunders C. Dehydration and the dying patient. *Pain Symptom Manage* 1995;10(3):192-7.
23. Byock I. Patient refusal of nutrition and hydration: Walking the ever-finer line. *American Journal of Hospice and Palliative Care* Mar/Apr 1995:8-13.
24. Hall JK. Caring for corpses or killing patients? *Nurs Manage* 1994;25(10):81-9.
25. Sullivan RJ, Jr. Accepting death without artificial nutrition or hydration. *Journal of General Internal Medicine* 1993;8:220-3.

See **www.hardchoices.com** for links to endnotes.

26. Holden CM. Nutrition and hydration in the terminally ill cancer patient: The nurse's role in helping patients and families cope. *Hospice Journal* 1993;9(2/3):15-35.

27. Andrews M, Smith SA, Tischer JF. Dehydration in terminally ill patients: Is it appropriate palliative care? *Postgrad Med* 1993;93:201-8.

28. Printz LA. Terminal dehydration, A compassionate treatment. *Arch Intern Med* 1992;152:697-700.

29. American Dietetic Association. Position of the American Dietetic Association: Issues in feeding the terminally ill adult. *J Am Dietetic Assoc* 1992;92:996-1005.

30. Lamerton R. Dehydration in dying patients. *Lancet* 1991;337:981-2.

31. Musgrave CF. Terminal dehydration: To give or not to give intravenous fluids? *Cancer Nursing* 1990;13:62-6.

32. Fugh-Berman A. Feeding the comatose patient: Procedures create major medical problems. *The Washington Post*, June 26, 1990.

33. Schmitz P, O'Brien M. Observations on nutrition and hydration in dying patients. In *By No Extraordinary Means,* ed. by Joanne Lynn. Bloomington: Indiana Univ. Press, 1989: 29-38.

34. Quill TE. Utilization of nasogastric tubes in a group of chronically ill, elderly patients in a community hospital. *Archives of Internal Medicine* 1989;149:1937-41.

35. Zerwekh JV. The dehydration question. *Nursing83* Jan 1983: 47-51.

36. Oliver D. Terminal dehydration (letter). *Lancet* 1984;2(8403):631.

37. Huffman IL, Dunn GP. The paradox of hydration in advanced terminal illness. *Journal of the American College of Surgeons* 2002;194:835-9.

38. Ahronheim JC. Nutrition and hydration in the terminal patient. *Clinics in Geriatric Medicine* 1996;12:379-91.

39. Casarett D et al. Appropriate use of artificial nutrition and hydration—fundamental principles and recommendations. *NEJM* 2005;353(24):2607-12.

40. Dy SM. Enteral and parenteral nutrition in terminally ill cancer patients: A review of the literature. *AJHPM* 2006;23:369-77.

41. Miyashita M et al. Physician and nurse attitudes toward artificial hydration for terminally ill cancer patients in Japan: Results of 2 nationwide surveys. *AJHPM* 2007;24:383.

42. Leff B et al. Discontinuing feeding tubes in a community nursing home. *Gerontologist* 1994;34:130-3.

43. Institute of Medical Ethics Working Party on the Ethics of Prolonging Life and Assisting Death. Withdrawal of life support from patients in a persistent vegetative state. *Lancet* 1990;337:96-8.

44. Ahronheim JC, Gasner MR. The sloganism of starvation. *Lancet* 1990;335:278-80.

45. Curtis E. Harris, who is both a physician and a lawyer, states "I do not consider the provision of food and water to be the medical treatment of a disease. Provision of food and water is normal or ordinary supportive care." Harris CE, Orr RD. The PVS debate: Even evangelical doctors may differ on this crucial issue. *Today's Christian Doctor* (published by the Christian Medical & Dental Society) 1999;30(1):8-13.

46. Former Surgeon General C. Everett Koop, along with the Association of American Physicians and Surgeons filed papers arguing against withdrawal of the feeding tube. "The clear object of the petition here is to end the life of Ms. Cruzan, an intent which is inimical to the very nature of medicine." Brief for the Assoc. of Am. Physicians and Surgeons. *Cruzan v. Director of Missouri Department of Health*, 497 U.S. 261(1990)(No. 88-1503).

47. Dr. Robert Orr says, that the withdrawal of artificial feeding in a permanently non-responsive patient . . . "is not killing. The discontinuation of a feeding tube in [a case like this] is an acknowledgment that the person is not going to recover, and a resignation to his death." see Harris, Orr, note 45 above.

48. "By definition, a patient in an irreversible coma cannot eat and swallow and thus will die of that pathology in a short time unless life-prolonging devices are utilized to circumvent the pathology. Withholding artificial hydration and nutrition from a patient in an irreversible coma does not introduce a new fatal pathology; rather it allows an already existing fatal pathology to take its natural course." Father Kevin O'Rourke, The AMA statement on tube feeding: An ethical analysis. *America: The National Catholic Weekly* Nov 1986;22:321-4.

49. Gostin LO. Ethics, the Constitution, and the dying process: The case of Theresa Marie Schiavo. *JAMA.* 2005;293:2403-7.

50. Caplan AL, McCartney JJ, Sisti DA, eds. *The Case of Terri Schiavo: Ethics at the End of Life,* Amherst, NY: Prometheus Books: 2006.

See **www.hardchoices.com** for links to endnotes.

51. Wolf-Klein G. Conceptualizing Alzheimer's Disease as a terminal medical illness, *AJHPM* 2007;24(1):77-82.

52. Volicer L; et al. Eating difficulties in patients with probable dementia of the Alzheimer type. *Journal of Geriatric Psychiatry and Neurology* 1989;2188-95.

53. Peck A, Cohen CE, Mulvihill MN. Long-term enteral feeding of aged demented nursing home patients. *JAGS* 1990;38:1195-8.

54. Reisberg B et al. The global deterioration scale for assessment of primary degenerative dementia. *American Journal of Psychiatry* 1982;139:1136-39.

55. Luchins DJ, Hanrahan P. What is appropriate health care for end-stage dementia? *JAGS* 1993;41:25-30.

56. Mitchell SL. A 93-year-old man with advanced dementia and eating problems, *JAMA.* 2007;298(21):2527-36.

57. Lo B, Dornbrand L. Guiding the hand that feeds. *NEJM* 1984;311:402-4.

58. Norberg A et al. Withdrawing feeding and withholding artificial nutrition from severely demented patients: Interviews with caregivers. *West J Nursing Research* 1987;9:348-56.

59. Post SG. Nutrition, hydration, and the demented elderly. *J Med Humanities* 1990;11:185-91.

60. Goldstein MK. Long-term enteral feeding: The British view. *JAGS* 1991;39:732.

61. Meyers RM, Grodin MA. Decisionmaking regarding the initiation of tube feedings in the severely demented elderly: A review. *JAGS* 1991;39:526-31.

62. Gillick M. Rethinking the role of tube feeding in patients with advanced dementia, *NEJM* 2000;342(3):206-10.

63. Finucane T, Christmas C, Travis K. Tube feeding in patients with advanced dementia: A review of the evidence. *JAMA* 282(14):1365-1370, Oct. 13, 1999.

64. Post S. Tube feeding and advanced progressive dementia. *Hastings Center Report* 2001;31(1):36-42.

65. Lynn Joanne, Harrold Joan. *Handbook for Mortals: Guidance for People Facing Serious Illness.* New York: Oxford University Press, 1999: 130-133.

66. Meier DE et al. High short-term mortality in hospitalized patients with advanced dementia: Lack of benefit of tube feeding. *Archives of Internal Medicine* 2001;161:594-9.

67. Hurley AC, Volicer L. Alzheimer disease: "It's okay, Mama, if you want to go, it's okay: Use of a feeding tube." *JAMA* 2002;288:2324-31.

68. Lyder CH. Pressure ulcer prevention and management. *JAMA* 2003;289:223-6.

69. Murphy LM, Lipman TO. Endoscopic gastrostomy does not prolong survival in patients with dementia. *Archives of Internal Medicine* 2003;163:1351-3.

70. Mitchell S et al. Clinical and organizational factors associated with feeding tube use among nursing home residents with advanced cognitive impairment. *JAMA* 2003;290:73-80.

71. Lacey D. Tube feeding, antibiotics, and hospitalization of nursing home residents with end-stage dementia: Perceptions of key medical decision-makers. *American Journal Alzheimer's Disease and Other Dementias* 2005:20:211.

72. Pasman HRW et al. Discomfort in nursing home patients with severe dementia in whom artificial nutrition and hydration is forgone. *Archives of Internal Medicine* 2005;165:1729-35.

73. Hoffer LJ. Tube feeding in advanced dementia: the metabolic perspective. *BMJ* 2006;333:1214-15.

74. Mitchell SL et al. A decision aid for long-term tube feeding in cognitively impaired older persons. *JAGS* 2001;49(3):313-16.

75. Monteleoni C, Clark E. Using rapid-cycle quality improvement methodology to reduce feeding tubes in patients with advanced dementia: before and after study. *BMJ* 2004;329:491-4.

76. Simmons SF. Prevention of unintentional weight loss in nursing home residents: A controlled trial of feeding assistance. *JAGS* 2008;56(8):1466-73.

77. DeLegge MH. Tube feeding in patients with dementia: where are we? *Nutrition in Clinical Practice* 2009;24:214.

78. Miller SC et al. Hospice enrollment and hospitalization of dying nursing home patients. *American Journal of Medicine* 2001;111(1):38-44.

79. Hanson LC, Ersek M. Meeting palliative care needs in post-acute care settings: "To help them live until they die." *JAMA* 2006;295:681-6.

80. Munn JC et al. Is hospice associated with improved end-of-care in nursing homes and assisted living facilities? *JAGS* 2006;54:490-5.

81. Lynn; Harrold, *Handbook for Mortals.* 1999: 1-14.

See **www.hardchoices.com** for links to endnotes.

82. National Hospice and Palliative Care Organization. www.caringinfo.org.

83. Berry ZS, Lynn J. Hospice medicine. *JAMA* 1993;270:221-2.

84. Callahan, Daniel. *The Troubled Dream of Life: In Search of a Peaceful Death.* New York: Simon & Schuster, 1993: 201-202.

85. Morrison RS, Siu A. Survival in end-stage dementia following acute illness. *JAMA* 2000;284:47-52.

86. Riesenberg D. Hospital care of patients with dementia. *JAMA* 2000;284(1):47-52.

87. Volicer BJ et al. Predicting short-term survival for patients with advanced Alzheimer's disease. *JAGS* 1993;41:535-40.

88. Volicer L et al. Hospice approach to the treatment of patients with advanced dementia of the Alzheimer type. *JAMA* 1986;256:2210-13.

89. Volicer L et al. Impact of special care unit for patients with advanced Alzheimer's disease on patients' discomfort and costs. *JAGS* 1994;42:597-603.

90. Rhymes JA, McCullough LB. Nonaggressive management of the illnesses of severely demented patients: An ethical justification. *JAGS* 1994;42:686-7.

91. Mitchell SL et al. Dying with advanced dementia in the nursing home. *Archives of Internal Medicine* 2004;164:321-6.

92. Mitchell SL et al. Hospice care for patients with dementia. *Journal of Pain and Symptom Management* 2007;34(1):7-16.

93. American Academy of Pediatrics Committee on Bioethics and Committee on Hospital Care: Palliative Care for Children. *Pediatrics* 2000;106(2), reaffirmed Pediatrics 2007;119(2).

94. Wolfe J et al. Understanding of prognosis among parents of children who died of cancer: Impact on treatment goals and integration of palliative care. *JAMA* 2000;284:2469-75.

95. McCabe MA et al. Implications of the patient self-determination act: Guidelines for involving adolescents in medical decision making. *J Adolescent Health* 1996;19:319-24.

96. American Academy of Pediatrics Committee on Bioethics: Guidelines on forgoing life-sustaining medical treatment. *Pediatrics* 1994;93(3):532-6.

97. Fried TR, Gillick MR. Medical decision-making in the last six months of life: Choices about limitation of care. *JAGS* 1994;42:303-7.

98. Lipsky MS et al. The use of do-not-hospitalize orders by family physicians in Ohio. *The Journal of Family Practice* 1990;30:61-7.

99. Mitchell SL et al. Decisions to forgo hospitalization in advanced dementia: A nationwide study. *JAGS* 2007;55(3):432-8.

100. Jencks SF et al. Rehospitalizations among patients in the Medicare Fee-for-Service Program. *NEJM* 2009;360(14):1418-28.

101. Meier DE et al. High short-term mortality in hospitalized patients with advanced dementia. *Archives of Internal Medicine* 2001;161:594-9.

102. Naparstek, Belleruth. *Staying Well With Guided Imagery.* New York: Warner Books, 1994.

103. Ankrom M et al. Elective discontinuation of life-sustaining mechanical ventilation on a chronic ventilator unit. *JAGS*, 2001;49(11): 1549-54.

104. United States Renal Data System. USRDS 1997 (and 1998) annual data report. Bethesda, MD: Natl. Inst. of Health, Natl. Inst. of Diabetes and Digestive and Kidney Disease; 1997 (and 1998).

105. Renal Physicians Association and American Society of Nephrology. *Clinical Practice Guideline on Shared Decision-Making in the Appropriate Initiation of Withdrawal from Dialysis,* Wash., DC: Feb. 2000.

106. Chen JH et al. Occurrence and treatment of suspected pneumonia in long-term care residents dying with advanced dementia, *JAGS* 2006;54(2):290-5.

107. van der Steen JT et al. Withholding or starting antibiotic treatment in patients with dementia and pneumonia: prediction of mortality with physician's judgment of illness severity and with specific prognostic models, *Medical Decision Making* 2005;25(2):210-21.

108. Azoulay D et al. Increasing opioid therapy and survival in a hospice, *JAGS* 2008;56(2):360-1.

109. Bottomley D, Hanks G. Subcutaneous midazolam infusion in palliative care. *Journal of Pain and Symptom Management* 1990;5:259-61.

110. Cernaianu A et al. Lorazepam and midazolam in the intensive care unit. *Critical Care Medicine* 1996;24:222-8.

111. Johanson G. Midazolam in terminal care. *Am J Hosp Pallia Care* Jan/Feb 1993: 13-14.

112. Mount B. Morphine drips, terminal sedation, and slow euthanasia: Definitions and facts, not anecdotes. *J Pallia Care* 1996;12(4):44-6.

See www.hardchoices.com for links to endnotes.

113. National Ethics Committee, Veterans Health Administration, The ethics of palliative sedation as a therapy of last resort, *AJHPM* 2007;23(6):483-91.

114. Stephenson J. The use of sedative drugs at the end of life in a UK hospice. *Pall Medicine* 2008;22:969-70.

115. Battin M. Terminal sedation: Pulling the sheet over our eyes. *Hastings Center Report* 2008;38(5):27-30.

116. Ely JW et al. The physician's decision to use tube feedings: The role of the family, the living will, and the Cruzan decision. *JAGS* 1992;40:471-5.

117. Fusgen I, Summa JD. How much sense is there in an attempt to resuscitate an aged person? *Gerontology* 1978;24:37.

118. Blackhall LJ. Must we always use CPR? *NEJM* 1987;317:1281-4.

119. Justice C. The natural death while not eating—A type of palliative care in Banaras, India, *J Pallia Care* 1995;11(1):38-42.

120. Callahan D. *The Troubled Dream of Life*, 1993: 81.

121. Lynn J. *By No Extraordinary Means: The Choice to Forgo Life-Sustaining Food and Water.* Bloomington: Indiana University Press, 1989.

122. Stoddard, Sandol. *The Hospice Movement: A Better Way of Caring for the Dying.* New York: Random House, Inc.,1991: xii.

123. Sonnenblick M, Friedlander Y, Steinberg A. Dissociation between the wishes of terminally ill parents and decisions of their offspring. *JAGS* 1993;41:599-604.

124. Thomasma DC. Reflections on the offspring's ethical role in decisions for incompetent patients: A response to Sonnenblick, et al. (editorial), *JAGS* 1993;41:684-6.

125. Ahronheim JC. State practice variations in the use of tube feeding for nursing home residents with severe cognitive impairment. *JAGS* 2001;49:148–52.

126. Mitchell SL. Nursing home characteristics associated with tube feeding in advanced cognitive impairment, *JAGS* 2003;51:75-9.

127. Kunin J. Withholding artificial feeding from the severely demented: merciful or immoral? Contrasts between secular and Jewish perspectives. *J Med Ethics* 2003;29:208-12.

128. Clarfield AM et al. Enteral feeding in end-stage dementia: A comparison of religious, ethnic, and national differences in Canada and Israel. *J of Gerontology* 2006;61A(6):621-7.

129. Wolfson C et al. A reevaluation of the duration of survival after onset of dementia. *NEJM* 2001;344(15):1111-6.

130. Rinpoche, Sogyal. *The Tibetan Book of Living and Dying.* New York: Harper,1992:34-35.

131. Koch KA, Rodeffer HD, Wears RL. Changing patterns of terminal care management in an intensive care unit. *Crit Care Med* 1994;22:233-43.

132. Callahan, D. *The Troubled Dream of Life*, 1993:149, 151

133. Becker, Ernest. *The Denial of Death.* New York:The Free Press, 1973.

134. Singh, Kathleen Diane. *The Grace in Dying: how we are transformed spiritually as we die.* New York: HarperCollins, 1998.

135. Callahan D. Death: "The distinguished thing." *Hastings Center Report* 2005;35(6):S5-S8.

136. Rinpoche, S. *The Tibetan Book of Living and Dying*, 33.

137. Psalms 103:14-16.

138. Dunn, Hank. *Light in the Shadows: Meditations While Living with a Life-Threatening Illness, 2nd Ed.*, 2005, p. 67.

139. Frankl, Viktor. *Man's Search for Meaning*, New York: Washington Square Press,1984: 90.

140. Nuland, Sherwin B. *How We Die: Reflections on Life's Final Chapter*, New York: Alfred A. Knopf,1993: 138-139.

141. Stoddard, S. *The Hospice Movement*, 204-205.

142. Rinpoche, S. *The Tibetan Book of Living and Dying*, 95.

143. Stoddard, S. *The Hospice Movement*, 211, 225.

144. Hillesum, Etty. *An Interrupted Life and Letters from Westerbork.* New York: Henry Holt & Co., 1981: 155.

145. Niebuhr, Reinhold. "The Serenity Prayer" (1934), quoted in *Familiar Quotations, 16th Edition*, edited by John Bartlett, Justin Kaplan, Boston: Little, Brown and Company, 1992: 684.

146. Quoted in: Petersen, David. Where the Phantoms Brood and Mourn. *Backpacker*, 1993;21:40-48.

147. Siegel, Bernie (interview). *Laughing Matters*. 1990;6(4):127-39.